# 7 WEEKS
# TO 100
# PUSH-UPS

# 7 WEEKS TO 100 PUSH-UPS

Strengthen and Sculpt Your Arms, Abs, Chest, Back, and
Glutes by Training to Do 100 Consecutive Push-Ups

**STEVE SPEIRS**

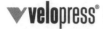

an imprint of Ulysses Press
PO Box 3440
Berkeley, CA 94703
www.velopress.com

ISBN: 978-1-64604-608-9
Library of Congress Control Number: 2023947121

Printed in the United States
10 9 8 7 6 5 4 3 2 1

Project editor: Brian McLendon
Managing editor: Claire Chun
Editor: Renee Rutledge
Proofreader: Joyce Wu
Index: Sayre Van Young
Design and layout: what!design @ whatweb.com
Interior photographs: © Andy Mogg except page 13 © Philip Date/shutterstock.com, page 42 © Jacqueline Hornyak/shutterstock.com, and page 45 © Romariolen/ shutterstock.com
Cover photograph: © Mike Manzano/istockphoto.com
Models: Micha Borodaev, Lily Chou, Lauren Harrison, Wellington Onyenwe

Please Note

This book has been written and published strictly for informational purposes, and in no way should be used as a substitute for consultation with health care professionals. You should not consider educational material herein to be the practice of medicine or to replace consultation with a physician or other medical practitioner. The author and publisher are providing you with information in this work so that you can have the knowledge and can choose, at your own risk, to act on that knowledge. The author and publisher also urge all readers to be aware of their health status and to consult health care professionals before beginning any health program.

To my wife, Ally, for her nonstop support, belief, and encouragement, and to my wonderful parents for always being there. *Diolch*

# CONTENTS

# Preface

Welcome to the exciting journey of transforming your upper-body strength and achieving the impressive milestone of performing 100 push-ups! This book, a reissue of *7 Weeks to 100 Push-Ups*, is designed to guide you step by step toward this notable feat. Whether you're a beginner looking to develop your strength or an experienced fitness enthusiast aiming for a new challenge, this program will provide you with the structure and guidance needed to reach your goals.

Since *7 Weeks to 100 Push-Ups* was released in 2009, numerous fitness fads have come and gone—everything from "as seen on TV" miracle devices to the current trend of track-everything apps and web-based systems. Push-ups are just as popular, and the seven-week plan just as effective, as they were 14 years ago.

I first dabbled with push-ups around 2007 to complement a marathon training plan I was following at the time. I enjoyed the simplicity of the exercise and the push-ups neatly added some much-needed variety to my typical run-only training regimen. Furthermore, coupled with a basic core workout routine, push-ups were an effective tool to help improve running economy and improve my race times.

Nowadays, at 57 years old, the majority of push-ups I perform are of the modified knee variety. Knee push-ups reduce the lifting load by about 50 percent but target the same muscles as the full push-up. I still run daily and enjoy racing everything from a 5-kilometer road race to 100-mile events on the trail, attributing some of my success to the humble push-up.

This book is for anyone looking to improve their upper-body and core strength. From the dad following the program at home with his children, to the high school teacher promoting the benefits of push-ups and consistent training to his students, *7 Weeks to 100 Push-Ups* can help reach your goals.

Over the years, people who have used this program have shared their success stories with me, including an 85-year-old man who "loves the program and loves his progress," a YouTuber following the program to help cope with depression, a high school senior using the program as preparation to pass an Army fitness test, and a mom of two little ones who has "never been this strong or fit."

Push-ups are a classic exercise that target multiple muscle groups, including the chest, shoulders, triceps, and core. They not only are a great measure of upper-body strength but also help improve stability, posture, and overall fitness. However, many individuals struggle to perform even a few push-ups, let alone reaching the milestone of 100. That's where this book comes in.

Over the next seven weeks, you'll embark on a progressive training program carefully designed to gradually increase your strength and endurance. The program takes into account your current fitness level and ensures that you make steady progress without overtaxing your body. By following the structured plan outlined in this book, you'll build the necessary strength and stamina to conquer the challenge of performing 100 consecutive push-ups.

Before we dive into the details of the program, let's address a common misconception. This book is not a magical shortcut to achieving 100 push-ups overnight. It requires commitment, consistency, and hard work. The journey will likely be challenging at times, but with dedication and perseverance, you'll witness remarkable improvements in your upper-body strength.

Throughout this book, you'll find valuable information and guidance on various aspects of push-up training. We'll explore proper form and technique, discuss common mistakes to avoid, and offer tips to maximize your progress. Additionally, we'll address the importance of warm-up exercises and recovery to ensure your body is primed for optimal performance.

One of the unique features of this program is its emphasis on progressive overload. Progressive overload can be defined as the gradual increase of stress placed upon the body during physical exercise. In a nutshell, this means steadily challenging your body to do more work over time. Progressive overload is vitally important to ensure your body keeps adapting and developing.

Instead of expecting you to immediately perform 100 push-ups, we'll break down the process into manageable steps. You'll start with an initial test to determine your base capability, and then gradually increase the intensity and volume of your workouts as you progress.

Remember, the key to success lies in consistent practice. You'll perform push-ups three times a week, with each session building upon the previous one. As you follow the program, you'll notice that your muscles adapt and grow stronger over time. Pushing your limits gradually will allow your body to adapt and prevent overuse injuries.

Beyond the physical aspects, this program is also about mental resilience. Pushing through the discomfort and fatigue will build your mental strength and discipline. Each successful push-up will not only strengthen your body but also boost your confidence and determination to reach the ultimate goal of 100 push-ups.

It's important to note that everyone's fitness journey is unique. Some individuals may progress faster, while others may take a bit longer to reach their goals. The key is to focus on your own progress and celebrate each milestone you achieve along the way. Try not to compare yourself to others but instead embrace the personal growth and transformation you experience throughout this program.

As you embark on this seven-week journey, remember to listen to your body. If you experience any pain or discomfort, it's crucial to modify or adapt the exercises accordingly. Always prioritize your safety and well-being.

I am excited to be your guide on this transformative journey. By the end of this program, you'll have not only achieved the remarkable milestone of 100 push-ups but also developed a strong foundation of upper-body strength that will enhance your overall fitness and well-being.

So, let's get started! Embrace the challenge, commit to the process, and witness the incredible changes that await you over the next seven weeks. Prepare to push your limits, redefine your strength, and ultimately, celebrate the accomplishment of 100 push-ups.

Best of luck on your journey!

Steve Speirs

October 2023

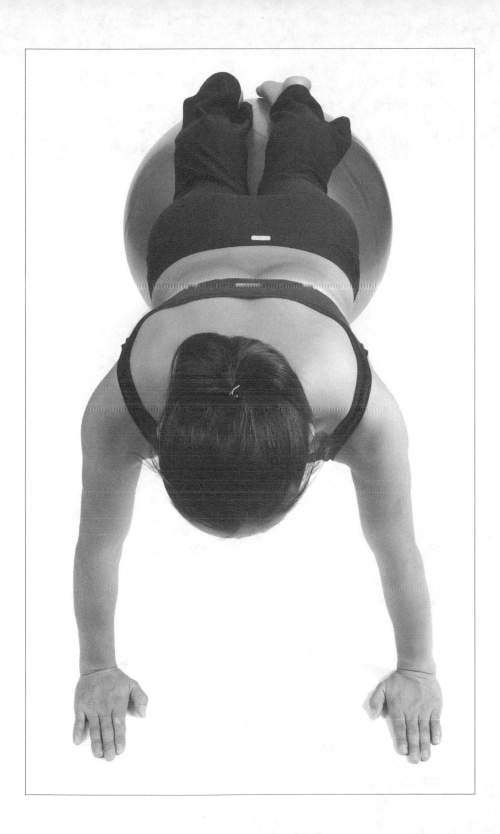

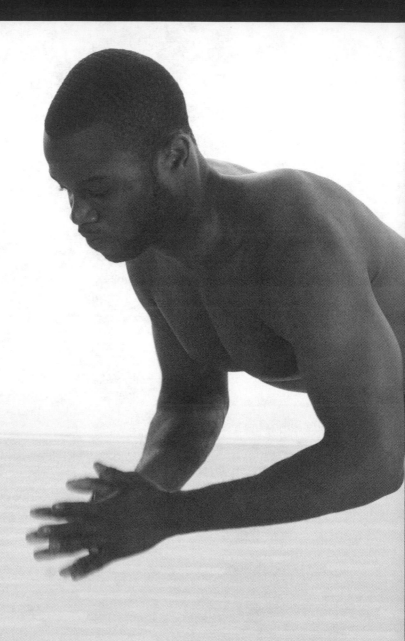

# PART 1:

# OVERVIEW

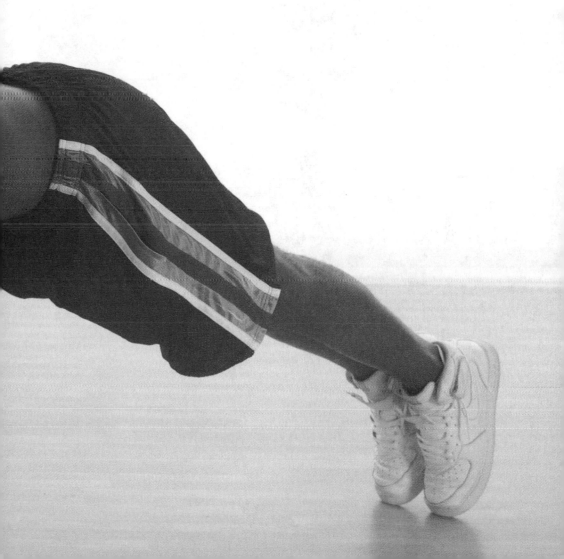

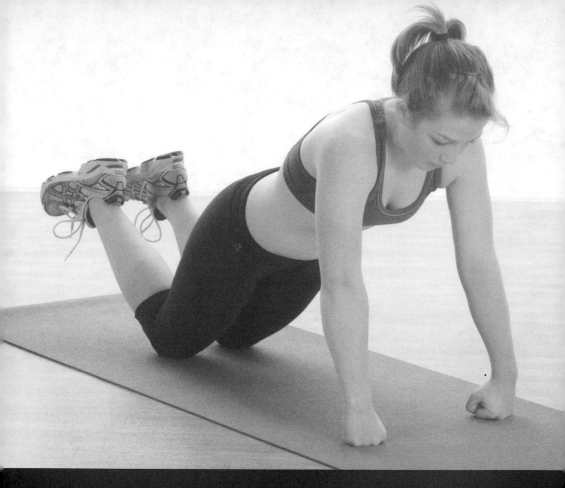

# INTRODUCTION

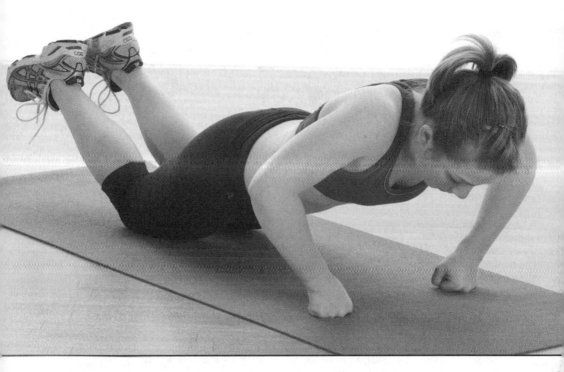

It's not easy staying in shape these days. Jobs are becoming more demanding, workweeks getting longer, family and friends taking up more and more of your precious free time but there are still only 24 hours in one day. And yet, in the same breath, we all want to have perfect bodies, too.

Keeping in shape, however, doesn't have to be time consuming nor inconvenient. Surprisingly, no matter how busy or complex your life is, you already have all the equipment you need for keeping fit and staying healthy.

More good news: There's no need to resign from the high-paying job, nor give up leisure time or family and friends. Push-ups are one of the most basic but rewarding all-around exercises you will find, and everyone from teenagers to older adults can benefit from doing them on a regular basis. The *7 Weeks to 100 Push-Ups* plan is an easy-to-follow, progressive training program designed to take you from your current fitness level to being able to complete 100 consecutive push-ups in just seven weeks.

The beauty of the plan is its simplicity; the workouts are easy to follow and no special training tools are required. Push-ups can be performed no matter where you are and, best of all, they are completely free—no expensive equipment or annual gym fees required!

The classic push-up has survived the test of time, and is the single most efficient exercise to simultaneously strengthen the chest, arms, deltoids, lower back, abs, and glutes. In simple terms, an equal effort is required to lower your body and raise it back up, and it's this controlled pace that works muscles as a team through three types of muscle-building resistance—concentric, eccentric, and isometric.

The benefits of push-ups are plentiful. Push-ups will improve muscular endurance within the upper body, strengthen both muscles and bones, create lean muscle mass that raises your metabolism, and of course, help keep you fit and healthy. If you're just looking to develop a great chest,

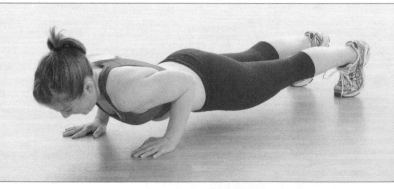

arms and shoulders, you could do much worse than follow along with the 100 Push-Ups plan. In addition, I guarantee you'll be surprised as your core strength goes through the roof, too!

Speaking as an aging but competitive runner, I'll be the first to admit I've neglected my upper-body strength in the past. However, in recent times, I realized the importance of developing muscular strength and endurance and as a result went in search of an easy-to-follow but challenging exercise regime.

The solution, I soon found, was the good old-fashioned push-up—a classic compound exercise to develop muscular endurance in the chest, shoulders, and arms. The logic I followed was simple: an increase in upper-body strength would help me become a better runner, and when the going got tough toward the end of a race, my overall strength would kick in and see me through to the finish line. I loved the fact that push-ups were such a straightforward exercise and could be performed literally anywhere with no special equipment. I took time to research various existing plans and workouts, and the rest, as they say, is history.

People lose up to 2 percent of muscle mass per year, eventually losing as much as 50 percent of muscle mass in the course of a lifetime. The effects of losing muscle mass include a decrease in strength, greater susceptibility to injury, and an increase in body fat. The good news, however, is regular exercise enlarges muscle fibers and will help stave off the decline by increasing the strength of muscle you have left. In fact, in many cases, strength training has been proven to reverse the loss of muscle mass and bone density due to aging.

I understand the most intimidating step is the first one. That's why this book also covers basic warm-up and stretching information and a variety of programs to suit all levels. In addition, you'll learn motivational tips and proper push-up technique, as well as be exposed to an array of alternative push-up styles if so required.

Still need proof that the *7 Weeks to 100 Push-Ups* plan is for you? Read the testimonials (which start on page 48) from real people who have completed 100 consecutive push-ups, and find out how a regular strength-training regime impacted their lives.

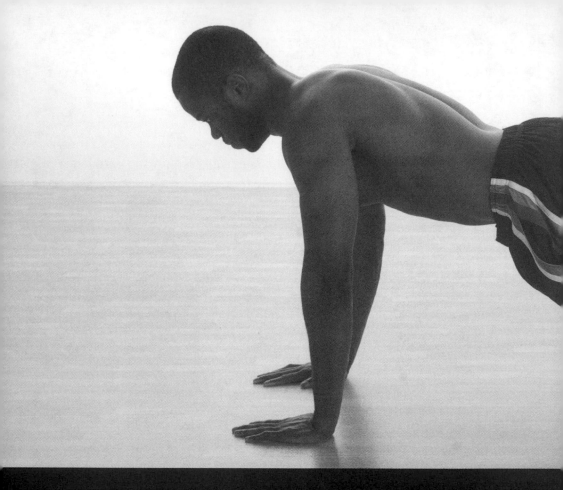

# ABOUT
# THE BOOK

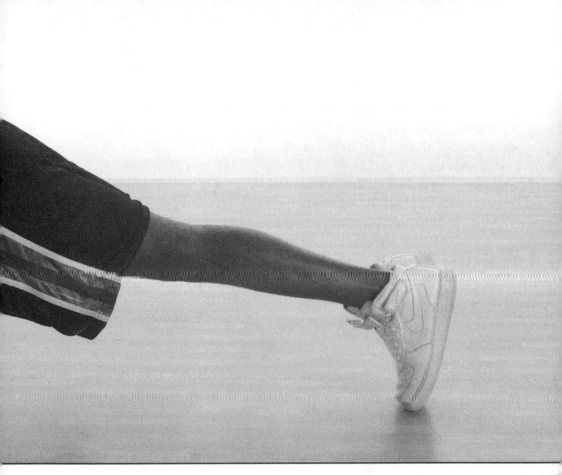

Fitness gains cannot be made without a concerted effort and a disciplined regime. After taking an initial test to determine your current fitness level, this book will guide you through a seven-week plan that is sure to set you on the road to a new, improved you. Hundreds of people just like yourself have already completed the program and been amazed at the results. All it takes is the will to succeed, steely determination, and a small time commitment each week.

This book contains four major sections, each with a specific goal. **PART 1** introduces the seven-week program, defines how to perform the perfect push-up, describes why push-ups are a fantastic exercise and details the benefits of following a structured training program. It also contains real-life testimonials from people who have successfully completed 100 consecutive push-ups, a list of frequently asked questions and steps to follow before embarking on the program.

**PART 2** outlines six different training plans—two ten-week programs aimed at beginners, two intermediate seven-week programs, and two seven-week programs for the advanced athlete. It also features an easy-to-follow maintenance plan so you can stay on top of your newfound strength.

**PART 3** details several alternative push-ups for those who have mastered the traditional push-up and are looking for more challenging versions.

Finally, the **APPENDIX** contains a log with which you can track your progress throughout the plan, a preliminary program for those not quite ready to tackle the seven-week challenge, and useful information on warming up and post-exercise stretching.

Sprinkled throughout the book are nuggets of push-ups trivia that highlight many of the great push-ups achievements of modern times.

Think 100 consecutive push-ups is tough? On October 5, 1965, Chuck Linster performed 6,006 consecutive push-ups. Robert Louis Knecht bested him on February 5, 1976, with 7,026. A year later (September 1, 1977), Henry C. Marshall did 7,650. Minoru Yoshida of Japan topped them all in October 1980, pumping out 10,507 push-ups in a row.

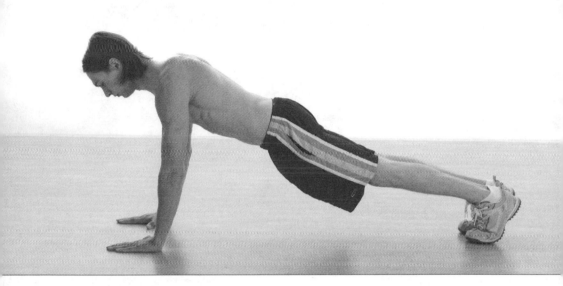

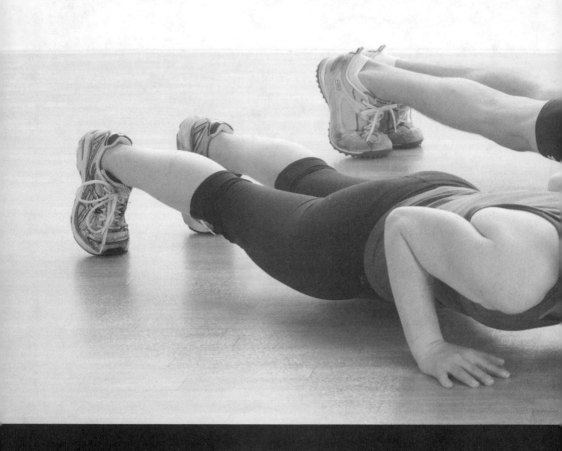

# WHAT IS A PUSH-UP?

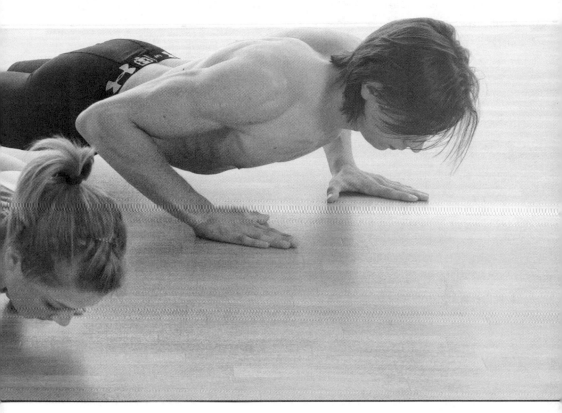

Are you haunted by memories of your P.E. teacher at school ordering you to the floor to "give me ten more!"? Push-ups don't have to be a chore and, in all honesty, they can be a lot of fun while also providing tremendous benefits. For this reason, the humble push-up is the most basic exercise used in civilian athletic training or physical education, and especially, in military physical training. Push-ups not only develop the upper body and the midsection as a whole, they also provide an effective cardio workout.

A push-up (or a "press-up" in British English) is a compound strength-training exercise that involves raising and lowering the body using the arms while face down in a prone, horizontal position. A compound exercise works several muscle groups at once, and includes movement around two or more joints. Most compound exercises build the basic strength that is needed to perform everyday activities, and push-ups are no exception. Push-ups are probably the most basic yet effective compound exercises known to man. Follow this seven-week plan and you'll be amazed how much easier routine tasks are to perform.

A quick search of the internet will reveal literally dozens of push-up variations. For the sake of simplicity, the *7 Weeks to 100 Push-Ups* plan focuses on the traditional push-up in which you assume a prone position with just your hands and feet in contact with the floor. More-advanced versions can be performed to target specific muscle groups, work different areas of the body, and provide a more challenging workout. See Part 3 (page 101) for full details.

*Note:* If you are currently unable to perform standard push-ups, turn to the preliminary program (page 166) for some alternatives. Performing these exercises will provide you with a base level of fitness so that you can progress with the seven-week training plan.

One final point definitely worth reiterating: A basic push-up does not require any equipment other than your own body weight, your arms, and a solid surface on which to support yourself. Push-ups can be performed anywhere you can find a firm surface and are therefore an excellent exercise for general upper-body strength. There are a whole host of push-up variations available to meet many different needs.

**Chung Kwung Ying of China did 2,750 "atomic" handstand push-ups on May 18, 1986. Also of China, six-year-old Lu Di managed 10,000 push-ups in three hours and twenty minutes on July 6, 2006.**

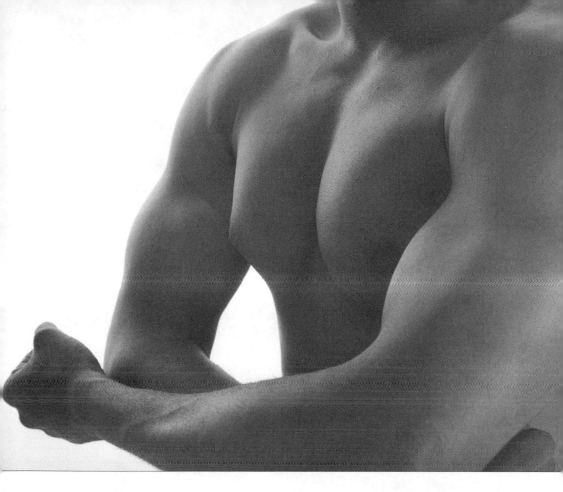

## The Muscles behind the Movement

One of the greatest benefits of push-ups (and strength training in general) is that of injury prevention. Nothing aids the skeletal structure more than strengthening the muscles and connective tissue around a specific area. This strengthening naturally occurs through regular training. From an aerobic standpoint, performing moderate to high sets of push-ups will provide an effective cardio workout, too. As an additional benefit, bone density is also improved, which vastly decreases the potential risk of injury in the specific body areas.

## IN THE BEGINNING

The origins of the push-up are not totally clear, although several known variations have been in existence for centuries. One school of thought is that the push-up as we know it today is a joining together of two popular yoga poses—downward-facing dog (*Adho Mukha Svanasana*) and upward-facing dog (*Urdhva Mukha Svanasana*). The roots of yoga can be traced back over 3,000 years.

Early examples of the exercise are also cited in Indian culture, where wrestlers would perform many hundreds of "Hindu push-up" repetitions. *Dands*, as they are more commonly known, build massive upper-body strength and endurance and have been used by champion Indian wrestlers for years. Legend has it that The Great Gama, the most successful Pehlwani wrestler in history, would perform upward of 2,000 *dands* each and every morning as part of a grueling training regime.

For the record, the phrase "push-up" was first recorded in the United States during the period from 1905 to 1910. Some 40 years later, the phrase "press-up" first appeared in the British lexicon.

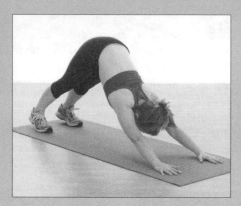

Downward-facing dog

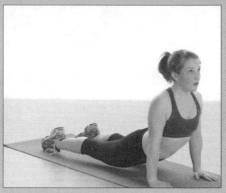

Upward-facing dog

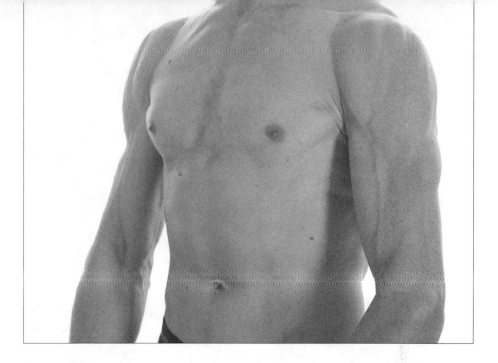

Push-ups are often considered difficult because the core stabilizer muscles of the hips and shoulders must be used to balance the body. Push-ups use all the muscles that make up the shoulder girdle and strengthen the smaller stabilizer muscles of the shoulder. The shoulder is the most mobile joint in the human body and is responsible for daily actions such as lifting, pushing, and pulling. Push-ups help to develop strength and flexibility for the wide range of motion required in the arms and hands. This strength and flexibility is especially important because the shoulder is extremely unstable and far more prone to dislocation and injury than other joints.

A number of other muscles are involved in a push-up:

**PECTORALS** The pectoralis major (commonly referred to as "pecs") is the fan-shaped muscle at the top-front area of the chest. Impressive chest development is usually the result of having well-defined pectoral muscles. The pectoralis major is responsible for three major actions—medially rotating the humerus (as in arm wrestling), flexing the humerus (as in lifting or throwing), and adducting the humerus (as in raising your arms to the sides of your body).

**TRICEPS** The triceps brachii (commonly referred to as "triceps"), the large muscle located on the back of the upper arm, is responsible for the action of straightening the arm. The triceps muscle makes up approximately 60 percent of the upper arm's muscle mass. *Note:* For increased triceps development, perform push-ups with a narrow hand position (pages 108, 112).

**DELTOIDS** The deltoid muscle is responsible for the much-coveted curved contour of the shoulder and is made up of three sections: front, side, and rear. Push-ups, although not a major contributor to deltoid development, are still an ancillary benefit to this muscle. The deltoid muscles take part in all movements of the upper arm, including lifting and rotating.

**SERRATUS ANTERIOR** The serratus anterior muscle originates on the surface of the upper ribs at the side of the chest and is largely responsible for the protraction of the shoulder blade. Traditional push-ups help to develop the serratus anterior, which is occasionally called the "boxer's muscle."

**ABS** The rectus abdominis muscle (commonly referred to as "abs") is the large, straight muscle at the front of the abdomen that supports the muscles of the spine. When performing push-ups, the lower back muscles contract to stabilize your body; this has a secondary benefit of stretching the abdominal muscles and developing core strength.

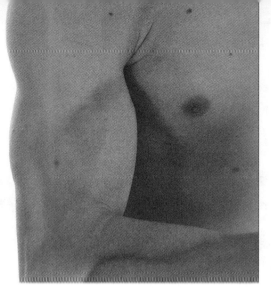

**THE** gluteus maximus (commonly referred to as "glutes") is the coarse muscle that makes up a large portion of the buttocks area and is largely responsible for maintaining the trunk in the erect posture.

**BICEPS** The biceps brachii (commonly referred to as "biceps"), the muscle located on the front of the upper arm, is responsible for forearm rotation and elbow flexion. However, biceps are not developed to any significant degree while performing traditional push-ups.

In a nutshell, push-ups give you more strength to carry out the activities you do every day. Lifting, carrying, moving, cleaning, gardening—these daily chores will all be so much easier to do as you work your way through the *7 Weeks to 100 Push-Ups* challenge.

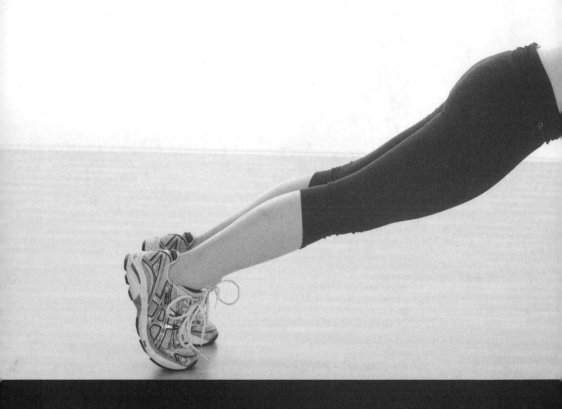

# WHY PUSH-UPS?

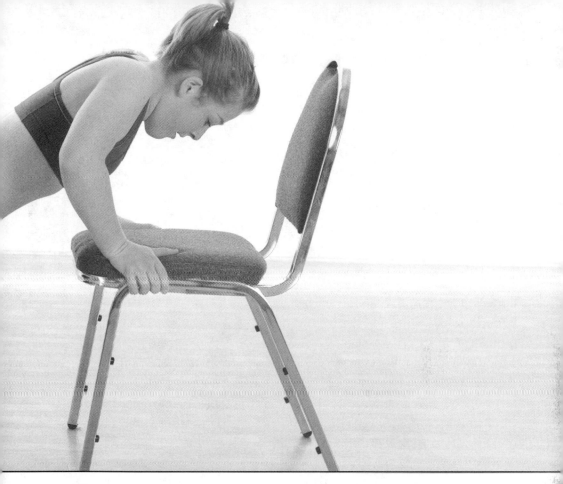

Push-ups are functional, multi-joint, multi-muscle movements that mimic the actions and movements we perform on an everyday basis. If you're already following a structured strength-training plan, you may question why you need to begin the seven-week push-ups challenge at all. Well, not only will your upper body see a marked increase in strength, you'll see big improvements in core stability and receive noticeable aerobic benefits, too. Quite simply, if you're looking for extra strength and stability and the ability to target specific muscle areas, push-ups are for you.

# Push-Ups in the Military

Push-ups are an integral part of military physical fitness and many military systems around the world train daily with the classic exercise. Most branches of the U.S. military service, including the Army, Air Force, Marines, and Navy, require push-ups on their physical fitness standards test.

There is arguably no better test of upper-body strength than the ability to perform push-ups, and this is probably the reason why special operations forces take pride in performing advanced versions of the

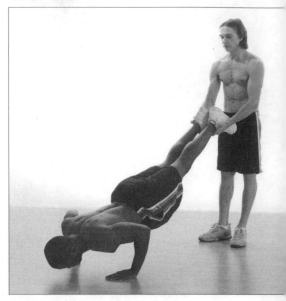

push-up to test their bodies. As an example, the tables below detail current U.S. Army standards for the number of push-ups performed within a two-minute period. How well do you stack up?

## U.S. Army Standards*

### PUSH-UPS MALE

| Age Group | 17–22 | 22–26 | 27–31 | 32–36 | 37–41 | 42–46 | 47–51 | 52–56 | 57–61 | 62+ |
|---|---|---|---|---|---|---|---|---|---|---|
| Maximum 100% | 71 | 75 | 77 | 75 | 73 | 66 | 59 | 56 | 54 | 50 |
| Minimum 60% | 42 | 40 | 39 | 36 | 34 | 31 | 25 | 20 | 18 | 16 |

### PUSH-UPS FEMALE

| Age Group | 17–22 | 22–26 | 27–31 | 32–36 | 37–41 | 42–46 | 47–51 | 52–56 | 57–61 | 62+ |
|---|---|---|---|---|---|---|---|---|---|---|
| Maximum 100% | 42 | 46 | 50 | 45 | 40 | 37 | 34 | 31 | 28 | 25 |
| Minimum 60% | 19 | 17 | 17 | 15 | 14 | 12 | 10 | 9 | 8 | 7 |

*performed within a two-minute period

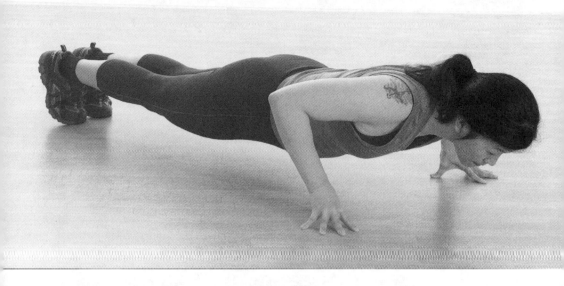

## Push-Ups in Sports and Film

A number of athletes in modern history have credited their phenomenal strength and success to the humble push-up. The great NFL player Herschel Walker, for one, never lifted weights and claimed push-ups were his only muscle-building exercise. Walker went on to win a Heisman Trophy and gained more than 13,000 yards in two professional football leagues. In 2006, Walker stated in a phone interview that he still performs 2,500 sit-ups and 1,500 push-ups every morning—a strict routine he has followed each day since high school. Boston Red Sox outfielder Ted Williams performed 50 to 100 fingertip push-ups every day.

Wrestling was once a royal national sport in India. Wrestlers born into the dying art of Kusti would rise daily at 5:30 a.m. to perform thousands of Hindu-style push-ups and squats, resulting in incredible amounts of strength and endurance. The Great Gama, billed as the most successful Pehlwani wrestler in history, would perform upward of 2,000 Hindu-style push-ups in a single workout. To this date he is the only wrestler in history to remain undefeated his whole life, with a career spanning more than 50 years.

Push-ups are a staple exercise for champion boxers around the world. Boxing legends like Rocky Marciano, Muhammad Ali, and George Foreman all did push-ups by the hundreds. In addition, Bruce Lee, a legendary Chinese martial artist, placed heavy emphasis on his arms and chest and attributed much of his upper-body strength to countless sets of push-ups. Lee is also famous for performing repetitions of two-finger push-ups using the thumb and index finger at the 1964 Long Beach International Karate Championships.

Bodybuilders, too, acknowledge the benefits of push-ups. On several occasions, 1970s champion bodybuilder Bill Pettis, famous for his 23¼-inch arms, would perform entire workouts consisting of 3,000 or more

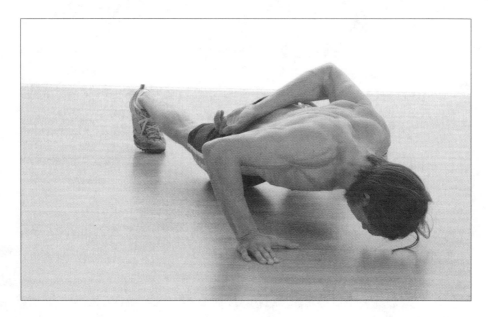

push-ups. The workouts would take at least five hours to complete. George Eiferman, a 1940s classic bodybuilder famous for his chest development, was well known for a grueling push-up workout in which he'd place both hands on raised benches to maximize the distance he could lower his torso. It's no coincidence his impressive chest development would rival many modern-day bodybuilders.

Hollywood has been known to utilize the push-up when creating enviable physiques. For the movie *G.I. Jane*, actress Demi Moore followed a grueling Navy SEAL training program made up of obstacle-course training, running, swimming, and of course, hundreds of push-ups. Moore is probably best remembered in *G.I. Jane* for her one-arm push-ups.

Actor Clint Eastwood would work out strenuously every day. Allegedly, when he was at the peak of his fitness, he would perform an impressive 1,000 push-ups a day.

## A PUSH-UP PHENOM

Great Britain's Paddy Doyle has held several records in the *Guinness Book of World Records* since 1987. On May 28, 1987, he did 4,100 push-ups with a 50-pound plate weight on his back. On February 12, 1990, he pumped out 2,521 one-arm push-ups in one hour; he would later do 8,794 one-arm push-ups in five hours on February 12, 1996. He managed 1,500,230 push-ups over the course of one year (October 1988–89). On November 8, 2007, he performed 1,940 push-ups using the back of his hands in one hour.

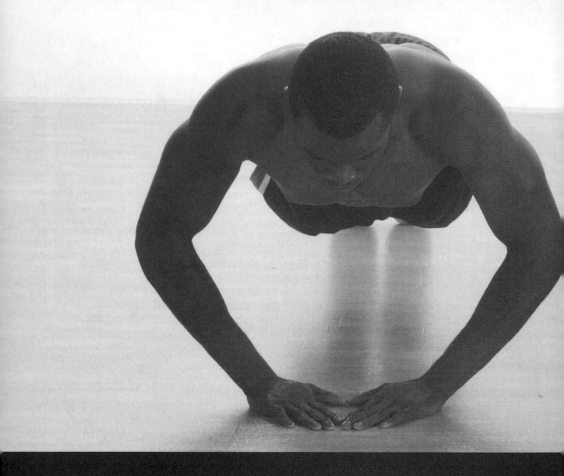

# FREQUENTLY ASKED QUESTIONS

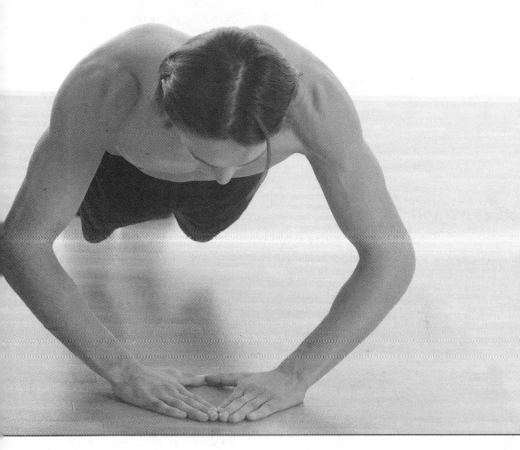

To help you gain the most from the *7 Weeks to 100 Push-Ups* program, I've assembled a list of answers to the 20 most commonly asked questions, covering topics such as correct form, workout frequency, weight loss, rest/recovery, and more. You'll also find suggestions for supplemental exercises, what changes to expect while following the plan, and what to do if you struggle with "traditional" push-ups.

# 1 Can I do push-ups every day instead of following the three-day-a-week plan?

No. It is very important to allow your body time to recover from the intense daily workouts. Muscle tissue is broken down during exercise but will rebuild itself during periods of rest and recovery. Working the muscles on consecutive days will hamper the rebuilding process and limit your progress. Remember, the body needs 48 hours to recover and adapt to the stress of strength training.

# 2 I've reached a plateau and can't do any more push-ups? What happened?

After making impressive strength gains early on in the program, occasionally your body will take a while to "catch up." Stick with the plan, trust in the numbers, and you'll soon be on your way to doing 100 push-ups. Also, ensure you breathe correctly during the workout. Holding your breath inhibits your ability to perform "good-form" push-ups and should be avoided.

# 3 My wrists hurt doing the push-ups. What should I do?

Try closing your hands and making a fist to perform the push-ups. This way your body weight ends up on your knuckles instead of your palms, thus avoiding the wrist extension motion. Please be sure to do this type of push-up on a padded mat, plush carpet, or even better, a folded towel.

# 4 Should my chest touch the floor on the down phase of the push-up?

Good form should put your chest within an inch or two of the floor. There is no specific need to touch the floor with your chest, but aim to form a 90-degree angle at your elbow joint.

# 5 How fast should I do the push-ups?

Push-ups should be performed in a slow, deliberate manner. Rather than bouncing up and down, it's important to maintain full control as you lower and raise your body. As a rough guide, each phase—both up and down—of a single push-up should take a couple of seconds.

**6** **What is the correct method for breathing during push-ups?**
It's important to breathe in during the descent and breathe out on the ascent. Make sure you don't hold your breath and make every effort to breathe rhythmically throughout the exercise.

**7** **What is the correct head position?**
Your head should be held in a neutral position—that is, not looking forward, up, or down at your navel. Traditional army push-ups have you looking forward, but in my opinion, this puts too much strain on your neck muscles.

**8** **Can I pause between push-ups if I begin to tire?**
Pausing for a short period of time to regain your composure is allowed, but make sure you rest in the "up" position. Do not lock your elbows, raise your butt, or allow your elbows to rest on the ground for assistance.

**9** **I'm unable to do one single traditional-style push-up. What can I do?**
Begin with the preliminary program (see page 166). Here you'll find push-up variations to suit everyone's current fitness level.

**10** **Will I lose weight if I follow the *7 Weeks to 100 Push-Ups* plan?**
Push-ups alone will burn some calories and do help increase muscle mass to some degree, which in turn takes more calories to maintain. However, push-ups by themselves are not the best way to lose weight—you really need to add an effective cardio training program to any type of strength-training plan if your main goal is weight loss.

## 11 My son/daughter is keen to take the challenge. Is the program safe for teenagers?

Absolutely! Actually, teenagers are very receptive to strength training and will make excellent progress by following the plan. However, please make sure your son/daughter is in good health, and if there are any doubts regarding their fitness, please seek medical advice before starting the challenge.

## 12 My arms tremble after I've completed my push-ups. Is this normal?

Yes. The "trembling" sensation in your arms is a sign of lactic acid build-up in your muscles—a sure sign of a strenuous workout. Stretching post-workout will help flush the lactic acid from your system and return the arms to their normal state. I've provided a number of stretches toward the rear of the book (see page 154).

## 13 What changes can I expect if I follow the plan?

As you work your way through the seven-week plan, you'll notice a dramatic increase in upper-body strength. In addition to the strength gains, you can expect to see muscular development in your chest, shoulders, and arms, although this usually takes a few weeks longer as the body works to synthesize the proteins that are used in muscle contractions.

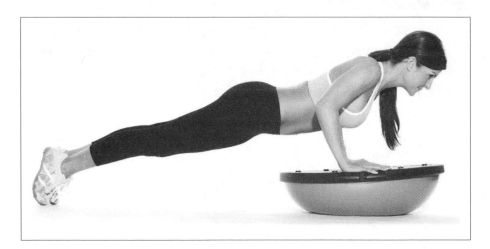

## 14 Can I use push-up bars?

People with weak wrists have reported some success using push-up bars instead of the traditional flat-palm-on-the-floor technique. However, with the extra height of the bars, there is a risk of lowering your chest too far and damaging connective tissues. The angle of your elbow joint should not become smaller than 45 degrees.

## 15 I'm still sore from a previous workout. Should I continue with the plan?

This is where you need to listen to your body. Is the pain general fatigue from the effort of a workout or did you do too much and cause damage to a muscle? If there's any doubt as to your ability to continue with the plan, stop immediately, take some time off, and seek medical advice.

## 16 Can I do other upper-body workouts on the same day as my push-ups?

It is fine to supplement your existing strength-training program with the 100 Push-Ups plan (or vice versa), but expect your performance to be slightly below par. Aim to rest a little between workouts, otherwise you may risk injuring a muscle or worse. A thorough warm-up and post-workout stretching regime is recommended.

## 17 The program states, "Rest 60 seconds between sets." What do I do while I'm resting?

It's completely up to you! Stand up, stretch, walk around, sip water, shake out your arms and shoulders. Just make sure you're ready to start again when the rest period is over.

# 18 My elbows hurt when I do the push-ups. What am I doing wrong?

Many people make the mistake of locking their elbows on the "up" phase of the push-up, which is considered to be very bad technique. At the top of the movement the arms should be almost straight, but be careful not to lock or snap them in place. Also, be sure to keep your elbows close to your body and not splayed out past your hands. If your form is good, you should feel a contraction in your triceps muscle. See page 62 for perfect push-up form.

# 19 When's the best time of day to do the program?

The best time of day to work out is very much a personal preference. Some people report they have the most energy first thing in the morning just after they wake up. Others, like me, prefer to work out in the late afternoon or evening. Your schedule may not allow you to exercise until last thing at night, but one great thing about push-ups is that they can be performed almost anywhere and at any time! Just make sure you allow enough time to warm up sufficiently and prepare your mind and body for the challenging workout ahead of you.

# 20 I tend to lose focus during workouts. How can I make push-ups more exciting?

Consider working out with a partner or, even better, in a group environment. For many people, workouts are definitely more fun when you're among friends, family, or work colleagues, and there is also the benefit of increased motivation and desire to do well. Another idea could be to perform push-ups to your favorite tunes. Some people prefer fast-tempo, upbeat music, while others prefer more relaxing, ambient music. Find a genre that works for you and have fun.

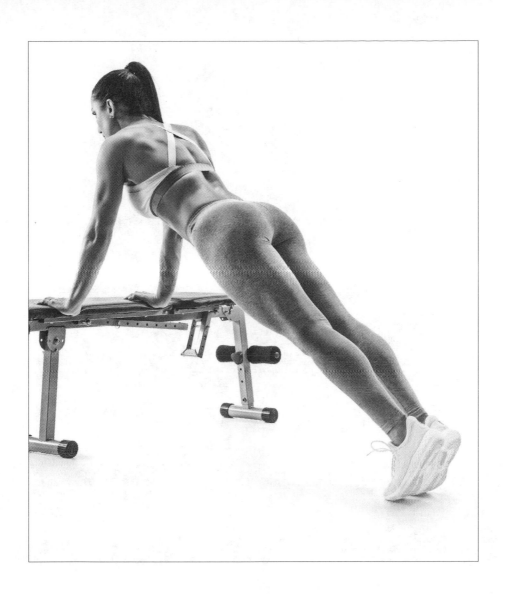

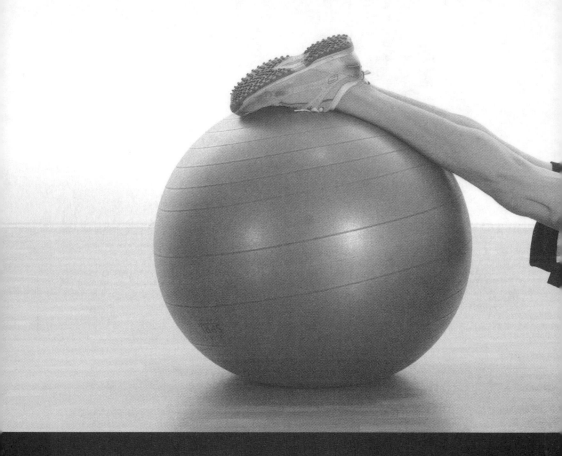

# TESTIMONIALS

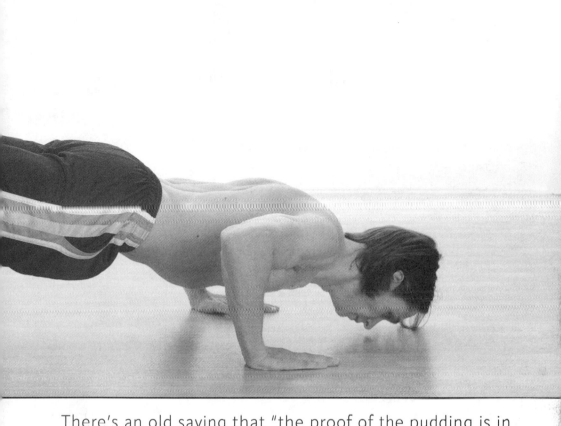

There's an old saying that "the proof of the pudding is in the eating," which basically means, to fully test something, you need to experience it. Don't just take my word for it. The following testimonials are genuine proof that with solid commitment, a positive mental attitude, and a modicum of self-discipline, the *7 Weeks to 100 Push-Ups* program, if followed correctly, actually works.

I ran into the 100 Push-Ups program and find it super great. I teach physical fitness at a small college and will use it to motivate my students. I also teach youth fitness, and the kids find the challenge to be the best I've given them. Especially with the kids, this program is really nice.

~Joe Coti
*Physical Education, Southwestern Michigan College*

Greetings from Mexico!

Thank you for the program, I find it easy and encouraging—but at the right measure! Not as easy as it looks and not as hard as to put off newcomers to the exercise. I completed the plan today and just wanted you to know how much good you have done! I am 47 and had done no push-ups for around 20 years—my initial test was 15, but after following the plan religiously, I today hit the magic 100 (103, actually). I will be continuing to do push-ups for fitness and strength; thanks for the inspiration.

~Steve Giles

I had my doubts even after week five, but when the time came to try the 100, I was able to do 105. The plan helped a lot with core strength and stability. Thanks for putting it out there!

~Cassie

Thank you for creating this program. Today, my 40th birthday, I achieved a goal I set 100 days ago: I did 100 push-ups! Actually, I did 101. I owe it to your excellent program. The first day I tried it, I could only do three push-ups. You've done a wonderful thing in creating this program. Thank you!

~Beverly Army Williams

I just wish this program had existed before I went off to basic training when I was in college. That would have been really helpful! The fact that I'm stronger now than I was in my 20s is astounding to me. Thanks again!

~Debbie Abrams

I tasted the success of 100 push-ups! I loved the challenge. The program framed my core beautifully and, because of that, has increased my performance as a runner. The future plan is to keep up the high number of push-ups in my cross-training routine.

~Holly Wert

I've always been one of those "lower-body strength" type guys (soccer player, sprinter, can leg press about eight times as much as I can bench press) and it's high time I found a program to get my top half in shape. Your program seems really well suited to cater to anyone's initial fitness level. Kudos on the great work!

~Dave Carlisle

I had to do 550 push-ups during the course of a two-hour red belt test for martial arts, and without your program, I would have failed!!!

~Nancy Milstone

**On September 13, 1987, Paul Lynch of Great Britain performed 32,573 push-ups in 24 hours; his record was beaten by Charles Servizio of the U.S., who completed 46,001 on April 24-25, 1993. Lynch later went on to finish 126 one-finger push-ups on April 21, 1992.**

I just started week three of the 100 Push-Ups program and I just can't believe that I am doing it. I am a 33-year-old man, but I have been sick all of my adult life with Crohn's Disease. During the sickness, I was weak, thin, and frail. With your program and my new healthy habits, my body is becoming…umm…muscular and toned. It is crazy. I was deathly sick four months ago and now…

Anyway, I appreciate the time that you spent on this program. Exercise always seemed too hard to get into. Where does a beginner start? Well, 100 Push-Ups is a good answer to that question!

~Daniel Berman

Steve, I just completed the final test. The program really works!

~Trail McFarland

I'm a 49-year-old mother of three elementary-school-age kids, working full time, who has been mourning my loss of fitness (used to swim and cycle hours/week). It was so nice to find something I could do at home when I had a chance without buying lots of equipment or staring at a home fitness DVD. I did push-ups from the knees because the arthritis in my MTPs makes them too painful from the toes. I started in mid-September and am now up to eight sets totaling 200 push-ups, with a final set of 100 push-ups, for a grand total of 300 push-ups, three times/week. Thanks!

*~Jan Baker*

I did my 100 attempt this morning and managed a very tough 102!!!!!! I am just so happy. I cannot believe I can do over 100 push-ups in one go! Not bad for a slightly overweight 42-year-old! :-) Thank you so much for the amazing program.

*~Dickie Armour*

Thanks for an inspiring program to help promote fitness. My wife and I have been trying to get in better shape, and I've chosen this as my next area of improvement. Thanks for the inspiration!

*~Grant Gardner*

My name is Season Gilbert. I am a runner and don't really work a lot on my upper-body strength so I thought this would be a great idea to get stronger. Never in a million years did I think that I would be able to do 100 push-ups...and there were a few training days that I didn't think I was going to make it through. But I stuck with it and am happy to say that today, in my seventh week, I did 100 consecutive push-ups! It wasn't easy, but I did it! We have now three other coworkers trying to complete the program, so thanks for the challenge!

*~Season Gilbert*

Took your challenge, and went from 53 to 104 during the six weeks. Thanks for the program—it did magic for my upper arms. ;)

*~Rune Pedersen*

I would like to thank you for the program. It has helped me become a lot stronger, and I am happy to say, 100 push-ups is easy! Eh, it's not really that easy, but from the 40 I could do before I started the program, 100 is really a lot!

~Curtis Sun

I'd just like to say that 100 Push-Ups is pretty amazing. Great routine that you cooked up. Very tough, but very doable.

~John Cool

My son and I are doing the challenge together—he's trying hard to beat the old man, but I'm keeping pace. Thanks for introducing this to us!

~J Faga & Son

There are six of us who are doing the 100 push-up challenge at work, and it's exciting! Amazing to see the progress we've made so far. Four of us are on week 5, and the other two are on week 3. :)

~Doug Adams

Just another person wanting to say thanks for the push! I started getting overweight since hitting 30, and now at 40, I definitely need to do something. The thing about exercise is, although you know you need to do it, it's the getting started that's difficult—that's where your program really helps. Despite a little break, I am noticing a big improvement already, despite starting as one of the un-fittest people. Anyway, thanks for the simple, easy-to-follow program!

~Tris

LOVE IT!!! Helping me get back to being as fit as I was in the Army!

~Joe Stern

Thanks so much for your challenge! This was a fantastic program, and people comment all the time about how muscular my arms look, thanks to your push-ups.

~Sagan Morrow

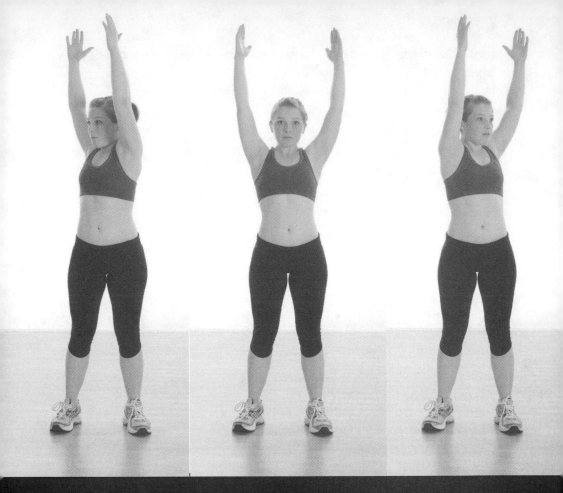

# BEFORE
# YOU BEGIN

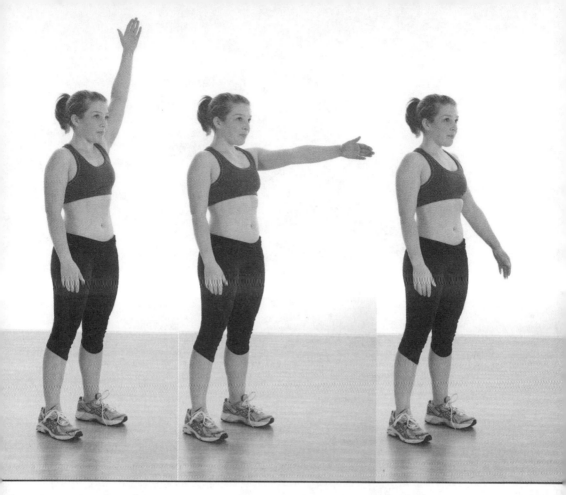

The plans in this book are suitable for all abilities, but before you commit to the challenge of the *7 Weeks to 100 Push-Ups* program, check in with your doctor, especially if it has been some time since you last undertook any kind of strength training. Find out what limitations you have, if any. The last thing you want is an injury that prevents you from reaching your goal.

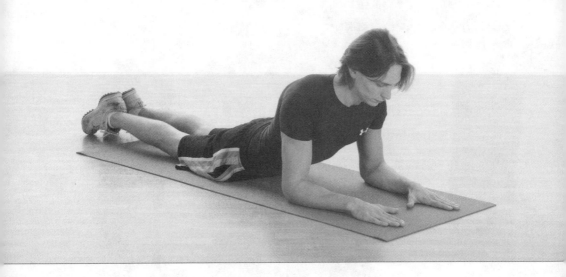

Once you've been given the all-clear, it's important to determine the correct level to start at. Take the initial test on page 60, and then make sure you follow the program that is designed for your current fitness level.

No special equipment is required to perform push-ups. Just make sure that the area in which you exercise is spacious and well ventilated. You'll also want to wear clothing that is comfortable and not too restrictive. Begin every workout in a well-hydrated state. Drink during the warm-up and sip from a water bottle during rest intervals, if required. If you find it difficult to motivate yourself to work out, why not recruit a few friends or family members to take the challenge with you?

# Injury Prevention

It's safe to say that nothing is more frustrating when you're training hard than encountering an injury. If you have any doubt as to your current ability to perform the *7 Weeks to 100 Push-Ups* program, please consult with your doctor or trained medical professional. A pre-existing injury may be aggravated if you dive into the initial test and begin the program without allowing enough time to heal properly. It is far more sensible to take a couple of recovery weeks now than to risk further injury and be sidelined for months.

As simple as this may sound, a good rule of thumb is to listen to your body. Nine times out of ten, you'll know if you're fit enough to start an intensive training program. Take heed of any warning signals Mother Nature throws your way.

As you work your way through the seven-week plan, expect to experience mild muscle soreness and fatigue, especially in the early stages of the program. It's very important to get in tune with your body and quickly learn the difference between "good pain" and "bad pain." Good pain can be the feeling of being "pumped" as your muscles fill with blood during exercise, or it can be the mild feeling of fatigue as the lactic acid burn sets in. Recognize these sensations and learn to thrive on them. Bad pain, on the other hand, is any sharp pain or spasm, or pain that moves quickly into the shoulders, arms, or hands—these are definite warning signs. DO NOT push through bad pain. Stop immediately, take time off, and seek medical advice from a doctor. It's much better to be safe than sorry!

Know when to push through any discomfort and know when to back off. Put your ego aside, take things slowly, and be ready and able to perform the next workout. Don't risk being sidelined for weeks with an easily avoided injury. Common problem areas include the wrists, shoulders, and elbows.

It is critical that you allow your body time to recover from these intense daily workouts. Muscle tissue is broken down during exercise and uses periods of rest and recovery to rebuild itself. Working the muscles on consecutive days will hamper the rebuilding process and limit your progress. Remember, the body needs 48 hours to recover and adapt to the stress of strength training. In addition, keep in mind that most injuries can be prevented by performing a thorough warm-up prior to exercise and a comprehensive stretching routine after your workout.

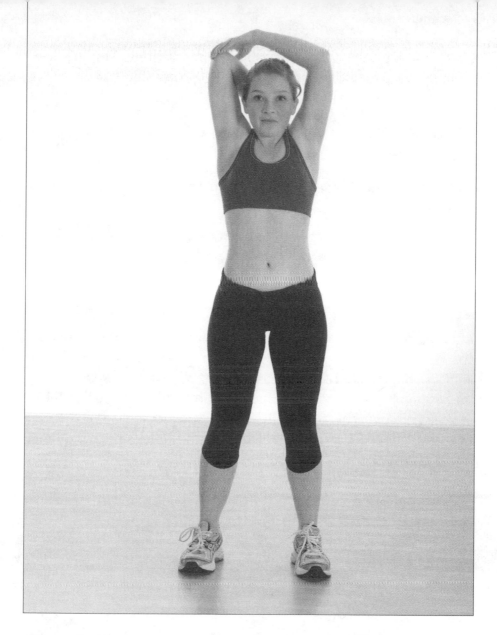

# Warming up and Stretching

A thorough warm-up is crucial to the success of your workout. For a variety of reasons, many people are tempted to rush right into the first set of push-ups, but please heed my advice and take the necessary time to raise your body temperature and heart and breathing rates. A proper warm-up mobilizes the joints and alerts the nerve-to-muscle pathways to prime your body for the activity it's about to undertake. Essentially, a warm-up gets the blood flowing to the muscle groups you are about to stress. My suggested warm-up (see page 140) only takes around 10 minutes, and is broken down into the following stages:

- **GENTLE MOBILITY** Easy movements that get your joints moving freely.

- **PULSE RAISER** Gentle, progressive, aerobic activity that starts the process of raising your heart rate.

- **SPECIFIC MOBILITY** Dynamic, exercise-specific movements that aid joint mobility.

- **FINAL PULSE RAISER** The last stage of preparing your heart rate and body temperature for exercise.

After each workout, remember to take time to stretch. This will lessen the chance of an injury and prepare your body for the next workout. Stretching immediately post-exercise when your muscles are still warm will yield the best results, including the greatest gains in flexibility. In addition, the muscles and connective tissues are more likely to respond favorably at this time, and there is less chance of a muscle strain. Key stretches can be found starting on page 154.

**August 30, 1998: Roy Berger of Canada performed 3,416 push-ups in one hour.**

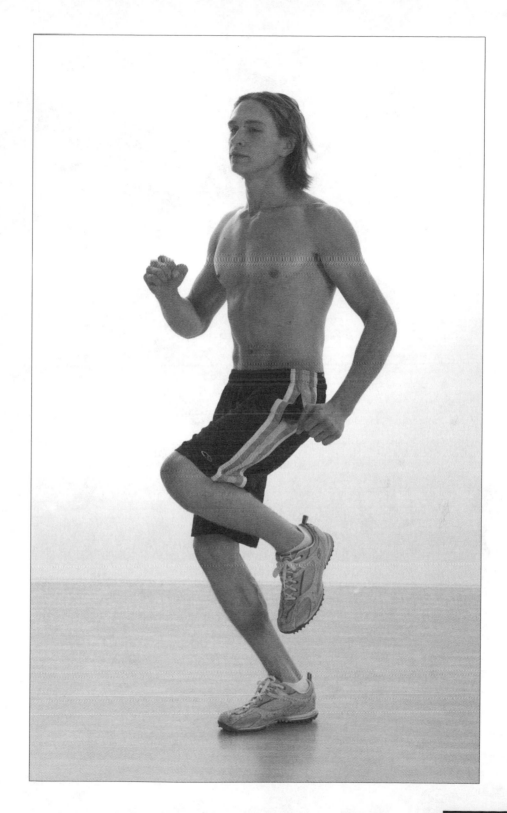

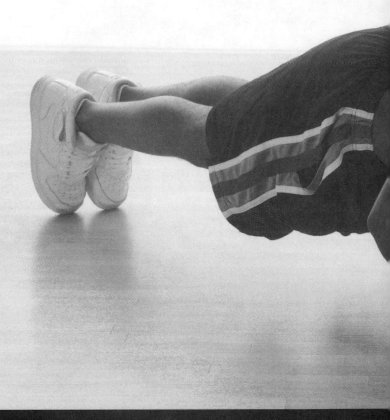

# INITIAL TEST

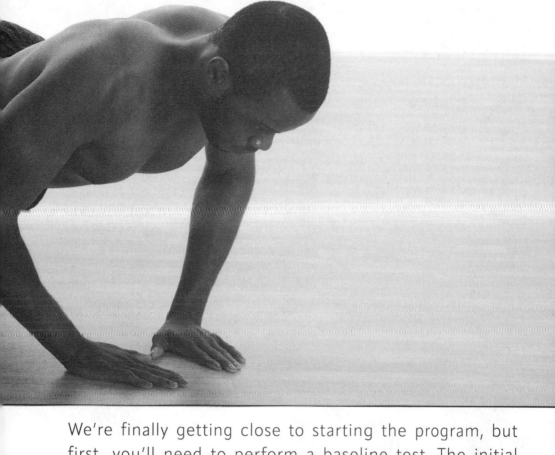

We're finally getting close to starting the program, but first, you'll need to perform a baseline test. The initial test is a great indicator of your current fitness level and will determine which plan to follow. Remember to always warm up before any exercise. Warming up reduces the risk of injury and prepares your muscles to do a push-up. You can actually lift/push/pull more if you go through a proper warm-up routine, as compared to diving straight into the exercises. A suggested warm-up routine can be found on page 140. Once you've warmed up, move on to the test.

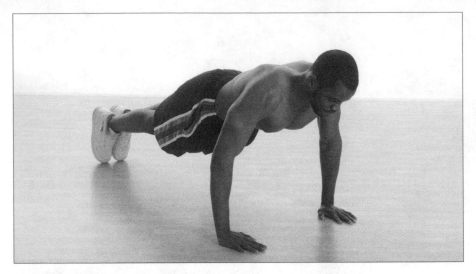

Starting position for the initial push-up test.

To begin, assume a prone position on the floor or other rigid surface that's able to support your body weight. Place your feet side by side with your toes curled toward your head so that the balls of your feet touch the ground. Place your hands on the floor approximately shoulder-width apart. Slightly wider than shoulder width is fine, too—whichever feels more comfortable. Make sure your elbows don't flare out past your hands. Maintain a straight line from your shoulders to your feet by keeping your abs tight. Do not raise your butt in the air or allow your back to sag to the ground.

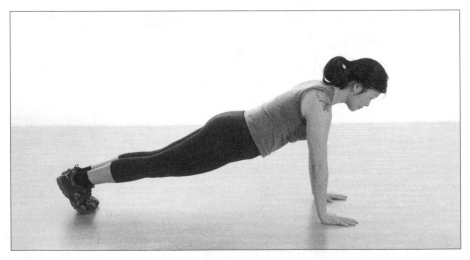

Maintain a straight line from your shoulders to your feet by keeping your abs tight.

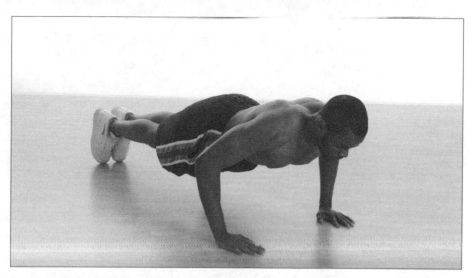
Push yourself up using your shoulders, chest, and triceps.

First, breathe in as you lower your torso to the ground, stopping when your elbows form a 90-degree angle and your chest is an inch or two from the ground. Keep your elbows close to your body for more resistance and keep your head facing forward. Try to keep the tip of your nose pointed directly ahead.

Next, breathe out as you push yourself up using your arms. Think of raising yourself by attempting to push the ground away from you. The power for the push will predominantly come from your shoulders and chest. You should also feel a contraction in your triceps (the muscle on the back of your upper arm). Continue the push until your arms are almost in a straight, but not locked, position.

Repeat the raising and lowering action of the exercise until you reach your maximum. Make sure you breathe in during the lowering phase and exhale on the raising phase. Holding your breath is to be avoided at all costs, as this will impair your ability to exercise and will probably cause dizziness and even blackouts. Also, do not continue past the pain barrier at this early stage in the program. No injuries, please!

Once you've done your maximum number of push-ups, the initial test is over. Hopefully, you surprised yourself with how many push-ups you could perform. If you didn't do as well as expected, don't worry—that's why you're following this program in the first place, right?

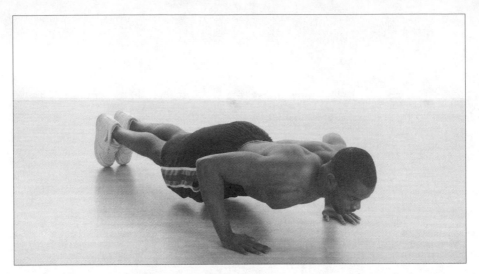

Stop when your elbows form a 90-degree angle and your chest is an inch or two from the ground.

Hopefully, you're still keen to start the seven-week program. Use the following guidelines to determine which plan you will be following:

| | |
|---|---|
| **0** | begin with the Preliminary Program (page 166) |
| **1–3** | follow the Beginner 1 plan (page 70) |
| **4–6** | follow the Beginner 2 plan (page 75) |
| **7–12** | follow the Intermediate 1 plan (page 80) |
| **13–20** | follow the Intermediate 2 plan (page 84) |
| **21–25** | follow the Advanced 1 plan (page 88) |
| **26+** | follow the Advanced 2 plan (page 92) |

To find out how you compare with other people of your gender and age, take a look at the test-result charts on the next page. The results don't really have any bearing on the seven-week plan, but they're useful to see how you stack up against friends, coworkers, and family members.

## MEN

|  | Under 30 | 30-39 | 40-49 | 50-59 | 60 and over |
|---|---|---|---|---|---|
| Excellent | 51+ | 47+ | 40+ | 33+ | 28+ |
| Very good | 41–50 | 37–46 | 31–39 | 25–32 | 21–27 |
| Good | 31–40 | 27–36 | 22–30 | 17–24 | 13–20 |
| Average | 21–30 | 17–26 | 13–21 | 9–16 | 5–12 |
| Poor | 0–20 | 0–16 | 0–12 | 0–8 | 0–4 |

## WOMEN

|  | Under 30 | 30-39 | 40-49 | 50-59 | 60 and over |
|---|---|---|---|---|---|
| Excellent | 41+ | 38+ | 31+ | 21+ | 16+ |
| Very good | 31–40 | 28–37 | 23–30 | 16–20 | 11–15 |
| Good | 21–30 | 19–27 | 15–22 | 11–15 | 6–10 |
| Average | 11–20 | 9–18 | 7–14 | 5–10 | 3–5 |
| Poor | 0–10 | 0–8 | 0–6 | 0–4 | 0–2 |

# PART 2:

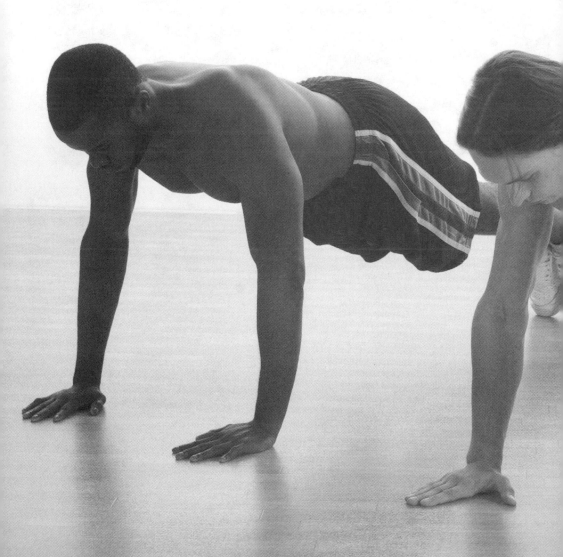

# THE PROGRAMS

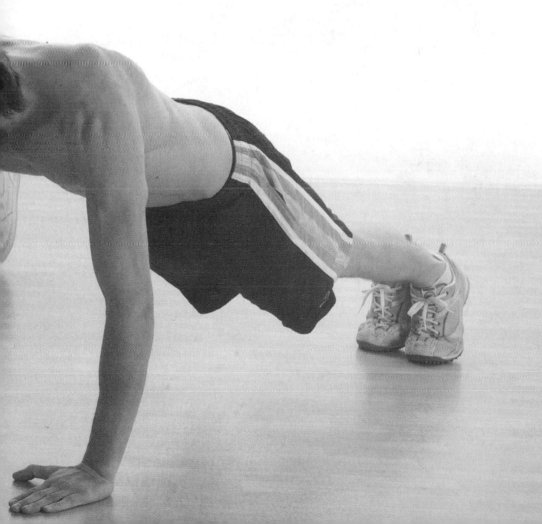

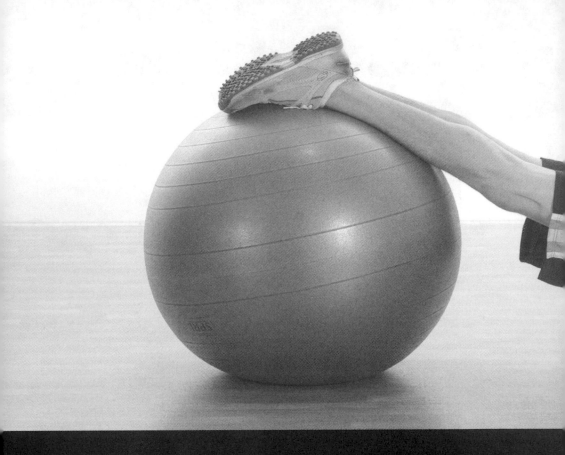

# THE 100 PUSH-UPS PROGRAMS

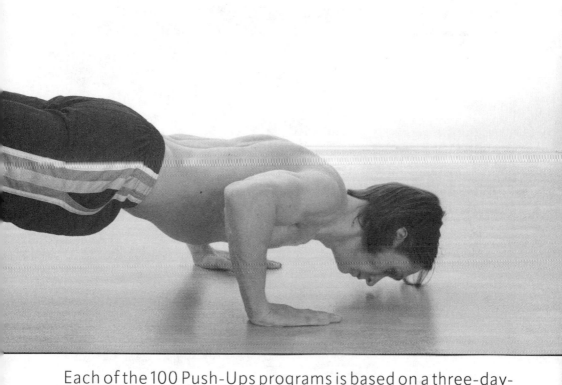

Each of the 100 Push-Ups programs is based on a three-day-a-week schedule. I would strongly recommend performing the exercises as a Monday–Wednesday–Friday routine, which tends to suit the majority of people embarking on a new workout regimen. However, the programs are flexible enough to be performed on any three days within a given seven-day period, leaving you free to choose your own personal start day. To help you chart your progress, I've provided push-up logs starting on page 182. If more than one person will be using this book, or if you anticipate trying out other push-up styles, make copies of the charts first.

*Note:* Rest and recovery are vital to the success of the programs and should be included as prescribed on the schedules.

## BEGINNER 1

| Week 1 | | SET 1 | SET 2 | SET 3 | SET 4 | SET 5 | SET 6 | SET 7 | SET 8 | |
|---|---|---|---|---|---|---|---|---|---|---|
| Monday | Warm up | 1 | 2 | 1 | 1 | 2+ | — | — | — | Stretch |
| Tuesday | | | | | Rest | | | | | |
| Wednesday | Warm up | 2 | 3 | 1 | 2 | 3+ | — | — | — | Stretch |
| Thursday | | | | | Rest | | | | | |
| Friday | Warm up | 3 | 4 | 3 | 3 | 4+ | — | — | — | Stretch |
| Saturday | | | | | Rest | | | | | |
| Sunday | | | | | Rest | | | | | |

| Week 2 | | SET 1 | SET 2 | SET 3 | SET 4 | SET 5 | SET 6 | SET 7 | SET 8 | |
|---|---|---|---|---|---|---|---|---|---|---|
| Monday | Warm up | 3 | 5 | 2 | 2 | 5+ | — | — | — | Stretch |
| Tuesday | | | | | Rest | | | | | |
| Wednesday | Warm up | 3 | 5 | 3 | 3 | 6+ | — | — | — | Stretch |
| Thursday | | | | | Rest | | | | | |
| Friday | Warm up | 4 | 5 | 5 | 5 | 7+ | — | — | — | Stretch |
| Saturday | | | | | Rest | | | | | |
| Sunday | | | | | Rest | | | | | |

**Rest 60 seconds between each SET (longer if required)**

**Remember to warm up and stretch! See pages 140–165.**

*Note:* Rest and recovery are vital to the success of the programs and should be included as prescribed on the schedules.

## BEGINNER 1

| Week 3 | | SET 1 | SET 2 | SET 3 | SET 4 | SET 5 | SET 6 | SET 7 | SET 8 | |
|---|---|---|---|---|---|---|---|---|---|---|
| Monday | Warm up | 4 | 6 | 4 | 4 | 8+ | — | — | — | Stretch |
| Tuesday | | | | | Rest | | | | | |
| Wednesday | Warm up | 5 | 7 | 6 | 6 | 9+ | — | — | — | Stretch |
| Thursday | | | | | Rest | | | | | |
| Friday | Warm up | 6 | 9 | 7 | 7 | 10+ | — | — | — | Stretch |
| Saturday | | | | | Rest | | | | | |
| Sunday | | | | | Rest | | | | | |

| Week 4 | | SET 1 | SET 2 | SET 3 | SET 4 | SET 5 | SET 6 | SET 7 | SET 8 | |
|---|---|---|---|---|---|---|---|---|---|---|
| Monday | Warm up | 8 | 10 | 7 | 7 | 12+ | — | — | — | Stretch |
| Tuesday | | | | | Rest | | | | | |
| Wednesday | Warm up | 8 | 10 | 8 | 8 | 14+ | — | — | — | Stretch |
| Thursday | | | | | Rest | | | | | |
| Friday | Warm up | 9 | 11 | 9 | 9 | 16+ | — | — | — | Stretch |
| Saturday | | | | | Rest | | | | | |
| Sunday | | | | | Rest | | | | | |

**Rest 60 seconds between each SET (longer if required)**

**Remember to warm up and stretch! See pages 140–165.**

*Note:* Rest and recovery are vital to the success of the programs and should be included as prescribed on the schedules.

## BEGINNER 1

| Week 5 | | SET 1 | SET 2 | SET 3 | SET 4 | SET 5 | SET 6 | SET 7 | SET 8 | |
|---|---|---|---|---|---|---|---|---|---|---|
| Monday | Warm up | 8 | 11 | 8 | 8 | 18+ | — | — | — | Stretch |
| Tuesday | Rest | | | | | | | | | |
| Wednesday | Warm up | 6 | 6 | 10 | 10 | 6 | 6 | 20+ | — | Stretch |
| Thursday | Rest | | | | | | | | | |
| Friday | Warm up | 7 | 7 | 12 | 12 | 6 | 6 | 24+ | — | Stretch |
| Saturday | Rest | | | | | | | | | |
| Sunday | Rest | | | | | | | | | |
| **Week 6** | | SET 1 | SET 2 | SET 3 | SET 4 | SET 5 | SET 6 | SET 7 | SET 8 | |
| Monday | Warm up | 8 | 13 | 8 | 8 | 26+ | — | — | — | Stretch |
| Tuesday | Rest | | | | | | | | | |
| Wednesday | Warm up | 6 | 6 | 10 | 10 | 7 | 7 | 7 | 28+ | Stretch |
| Thursday | Rest | | | | | | | | | |
| Friday | Warm up | 8 | 8 | 12 | 12 | 8 | 8 | 8 | 30+ | Stretch |
| Saturday | Rest | | | | | | | | | |
| Sunday | Rest | | | | | | | | | |

**Rest 60 seconds between each SET (longer if required)**

**Remember to warm up and stretch! See pages 140–165.**

*Note:* Rest and recovery are vital to the success of the programs and should be included as prescribed on the schedules.

## BEGINNER 1

| Week 7 | | SET 1 | SET 2 | SET 3 | SET 4 | SET 5 | SET 6 | SET 7 | SET 8 | |
|---|---|---|---|---|---|---|---|---|---|---|
| Monday | Warm up | 10 | 15 | 10 | 10 | 33+ | — | — | — | Stretch |
| Tuesday | Rest | | | | | | | | | |
| Wednesday | Warm up | 8 | 8 | 12 | 12 | 8 | 8 | 8 | 36+ | Stretch |
| Thursday | Rest | | | | | | | | | |
| Friday | Warm up | 10 | 10 | 14 | 14 | 10 | 10 | 10 | 40+ | Stretch |
| Saturday | Rest | | | | | | | | | |
| Sunday | Rest | | | | | | | | | |
| Week 8 | | SET 1 | SET 2 | SET 3 | SET 4 | SET 5 | SET 6 | SET 7 | SET 8 | |
| Monday | Warm up | 12 | 16 | 12 | 12 | 45+ | — | — | — | Stretch |
| Tuesday | Rest | | | | | | | | | |
| Wednesday | Warm up | 9 | 9 | 13 | 13 | 9 | 9 | 9 | 50+ | Stretch |
| Thursday | Rest | | | | | | | | | |
| Friday | Warm up | 11 | 11 | 15 | 15 | 11 | 11 | 11 | 55+ | Stretch |
| Saturday | Rest | | | | | | | | | |
| Sunday | Rest | | | | | | | | | |

**Rest 60 seconds between each SET (longer if required)**

**Remember to warm up and stretch! See pages 140–165.**

## BEGINNER 1

| Week 9 | | SET 1 | SET 2 | SET 3 | SET 4 | SET 5 | SET 6 | SET 7 | SET 8 | |
|---|---|---|---|---|---|---|---|---|---|---|
| Monday | Warm up | 13 | 18 | 13 | 13 | 50+ | — | — | — | Stretch |
| Tuesday | | | | | Rest | | | | | |
| Wednesday | Warm up | 10 | 10 | 15 | 15 | 10 | 10 | 10 | 55+ | Stretch |
| Thursday | | | | | Rest | | | | | |
| Friday | Warm up | 12 | 12 | 16 | 16 | 12 | 12 | 12 | 60+ | Stretch |
| Saturday | | | | | Rest | | | | | |
| Sunday | | | | | Rest | | | | | |
| Week 10 | | SET 1 | SET 2 | SET 3 | SET 4 | SET 5 | SET 6 | SET 7 | SET 8 | |
| Monday | Warm up | 15 | 20 | 15 | 15 | 50+ | — | — | — | Stretch |
| Tuesday | | | | | Rest | | | | | |
| Wednesday | Warm up | 12 | 12 | 16 | 16 | 13 | 13 | 13 | 55+ | Stretch |
| Thursday | | | | | Rest | | | | | |
| Friday | Warm up | 13 | 13 | 18 | 18 | 13 | 13 | 13 | 60+ | Stretch |
| Saturday | | | | | Rest | | | | | |
| Sunday | | | | | Rest | | | | | |

**Rest 60 seconds between each SET (longer if required)**

**Remember to warm up and stretch! See pages 140–165.**

*Note:* Rest and recovery are vital to the success of the programs and should be included as prescribed on the schedules.

## BEGINNER 2

| Week 1 | | SET 1 | SET 2 | SET 3 | SET 4 | SET 5 | SET 6 | SET 7 | SET 8 | |
|---|---|---|---|---|---|---|---|---|---|---|
| Monday | Warm up | 2 | 3 | 2 | 2 | 3+ | — | — | — | Stretch |
| Tuesday | Rest | | | | | | | | | |
| Wednesday | Warm up | 3 | 4 | 2 | 3 | 4+ | — | — | — | Stretch |
| Thursday | Rest | | | | | | | | | |
| Friday | Warm up | 4 | 5 | 4 | 4 | 5+ | — | — | — | Stretch |
| Saturday | Rest | | | | | | | | | |
| Sunday | Rest | | | | | | | | | |
| Week 2 | | SET 1 | SET 2 | SET 3 | SET 4 | SET 5 | SET 6 | SET 7 | SET 8 | |
| Monday | Warm up | 4 | 6 | 4 | 4 | 7+ | — | — | — | Stretch |
| Tuesday | Rest | | | | | | | | | |
| Wednesday | Warm up | 5 | 7 | 5 | 5 | 8+ | — | — | — | Stretch |
| Thursday | Rest | | | | | | | | | |
| Friday | Warm up | 6 | 8 | 6 | 6 | 9+ | — | — | — | Stretch |
| Saturday | Rest | | | | | | | | | |
| Sunday | Rest | | | | | | | | | |

**Rest 60 seconds between each SET (longer if required)**

**Remember to warm up and stretch! See pages 140–165.**

*Note:* Rest and recovery are vital to the success of the programs and should be included as prescribed on the schedules.

## BEGINNER 2

| Week 3 | | SET 1 | SET 2 | SET 3 | SET 4 | SET 5 | SET 6 | SET 7 | SET 8 | |
|---|---|---|---|---|---|---|---|---|---|---|
| Monday | Warm up | 6 | 8 | 6 | 6 | 9+ | — | | | Stretch |
| Tuesday | Rest | | | | | | | | | |
| Wednesday | Warm up | 7 | 10 | 8 | 8 | 11+ | — | — | — | Stretch |
| Thursday | Rest | | | | | | | | | |
| Friday | Warm up | 8 | 12 | 9 | 9 | 13+ | — | — | — | Stretch |
| Saturday | Rest | | | | | | | | | |
| Sunday | Rest | | | | | | | | | |
| Week 4 | | SET 1 | SET 2 | SET 3 | SET 4 | SET 5 | SET 6 | SET 7 | SET 8 | |
| Monday | Warm up | 9 | 12 | 9 | 9 | 15+ | — | — | — | Stretch |
| Tuesday | Rest | | | | | | | | | |
| Wednesday | Warm up | 10 | 13 | 10 | 10 | 17+ | — | — | — | Stretch |
| Thursday | Rest | | | | | | | | | |
| Friday | Warm up | 11 | 14 | 11 | 11 | 19+ | — | — | — | Stretch |
| Saturday | Rest | | | | | | | | | |
| Sunday | Rest | | | | | | | | | |
| | Rest 60 seconds between each SET (longer if required) | | | | | | | | | |
| | Remember to warm up and stretch! See pages 140–165. | | | | | | | | | |

**7 WEEKS TO 100 PUSH-UPS**

## BEGINNER 2

| Week 5 | | SET 1 | SET 2 | SET 3 | SET 4 | SET 5 | SET 6 | SET 7 | SET 8 | |
|---|---|---|---|---|---|---|---|---|---|---|
| Monday | Warm up | 9 | 14 | 10 | 10 | 20+ | — | — | — | Stretch |
| Tuesday | | | | | Rest | | | | | |
| Wednesday | Warm up | 7 | 7 | 12 | 12 | 7 | 7 | 25+ | — | Stretch |
| Thursday | | | | | Rest | | | | | |
| Friday | Warm up | 8 | 8 | 14 | 14 | 8 | 8 | 30+ | — | Stretch |
| Saturday | | | | | Rest | | | | | |
| Sunday | | | | | Rest | | | | | |

| Week 6 | | SET 1 | SET 2 | SET 3 | SET 4 | SET 5 | SET 6 | SET 7 | SET 8 | |
|---|---|---|---|---|---|---|---|---|---|---|
| Monday | Warm up | 10 | 15 | 10 | 10 | 30+ | — | — | — | Stretch |
| Tuesday | | | | | Rest | | | | | |
| Wednesday | Warm up | 8 | 8 | 12 | 12 | 9 | 9 | 9 | 35+ | Stretch |
| Thursday | | | | | Rest | | | | | |
| Friday | Warm up | 10 | 10 | 14 | 14 | 10 | 10 | 10 | 40+ | Stretch |
| Saturday | | | | | Rest | | | | | |
| Sunday | | | | | Rest | | | | | |

Rest 60 seconds between each SET (longer if required)

Remember to warm up and stretch! See pages 140–165.

*Note:* Rest and recovery are vital to the success of the programs and should be included as prescribed on the schedules.

## BEGINNER 2

| Week 7 | | SET 1 | SET 2 | SET 3 | SET 4 | SET 5 | SET 6 | SET 7 | SET 8 | |
|---|---|---|---|---|---|---|---|---|---|---|
| Monday | Warm up | 12 | 17 | 12 | 12 | 40+ | — | — | — | Stretch |
| Tuesday | | | | | Rest | | | | | |
| Wednesday | Warm up | 10 | 10 | 14 | 14 | 10 | 10 | 11 | 45+ | Stretch |
| Thursday | | | | | Rest | | | | | |
| Friday | Warm up | 12 | 12 | 16 | 16 | 12 | 12 | 12 | 50+ | Stretch |
| Saturday | | | | | Rest | | | | | |
| Sunday | | | | | Rest | | | | | |
| Week 8 | | SET 1 | SET 2 | SET 3 | SET 4 | SET 5 | SET 6 | SET 7 | SET 8 | |
| Monday | Warm up | 13 | 18 | 13 | 13 | 50+ | — | — | — | Stretch |
| Tuesday | | | | | Rest | | | | | |
| Wednesday | Warm up | 11 | 11 | 15 | 15 | 11 | 11 | 11 | 55+ | Stretch |
| Thursday | | | | | Rest | | | | | |
| Friday | Warm up | 13 | 13 | 17 | 17 | 13 | 13 | 13 | 60+ | Stretch |
| Saturday | | | | | Rest | | | | | |
| Sunday | | | | | Rest | | | | | |

**Rest 60 seconds between each SET (longer if required)**

**Remember to warm up and stretch! See pages 140–165.**

*Note:* Rest and recovery are vital to the success of the programs and should be included as prescribed on the schedules.

## BEGINNER 2

| Week 9 | | SET 1 | SET 2 | SET 3 | SET 4 | SET 5 | SET 6 | SET 7 | SET 8 | |
|---|---|---|---|---|---|---|---|---|---|---|
| Monday | Warm up | 14 | 20 | 14 | 14 | 50+ | — | — | — | Stretch |
| Tuesday | Rest | | | | | | | | | |
| Wednesday | Warm up | 12 | 12 | 17 | 17 | 12 | 12 | 12 | 55+ | Stretch |
| Thursday | Rest | | | | | | | | | |
| Friday | Warm up | 14 | 14 | 18 | 18 | 14 | 14 | 14 | 60+ | Stretch |
| Saturday | Rest | | | | | | | | | |
| Sunday | Rest | | | | | | | | | |

| Week 10 | | SET 1 | SET 2 | SET 3 | SET 4 | SET 5 | SET 6 | SET 7 | SET 8 | |
|---|---|---|---|---|---|---|---|---|---|---|
| Monday | Warm up | 16 | 24 | 16 | 16 | 50+ | — | — | — | Stretch |
| Tuesday | Rest | | | | | | | | | |
| Wednesday | Warm up | 14 | 14 | 19 | 19 | 14 | 14 | 14 | 55+ | Stretch |
| Thursday | Rest | | | | | | | | | |
| Friday | Warm up | 16 | 16 | 20 | 20 | 16 | 16 | 16 | 60+ | Stretch |
| Saturday | Rest | | | | | | | | | |
| Sunday | Rest | | | | | | | | | |

**Rest 60 seconds between each SET (longer if required)**

**Remember to warm up and stretch! See pages 140–165.**

## INTERMEDIATE 1

| Week 1 | | SET 1 | SET 2 | SET 3 | SET 4 | SET 5 | SET 6 | SET 7 | SET 8 | |
|---|---|---|---|---|---|---|---|---|---|---|
| Monday | Warm up | 4 | 6 | 4 | 4 | 5+ | — | — | — | Stretch |
| Tuesday | | | | | Rest | | | | | |
| Wednesday | Warm up | 6 | 8 | 6 | 6 | 7+ | — | — | — | Stretch |
| Thursday | | | | | Rest | | | | | |
| Friday | Warm up | 7 | 10 | 7 | 7 | 9+ | — | — | — | Stretch |
| Saturday | | | | | Rest | | | | | |
| Sunday | | | | | Rest | | | | | |

| Week 2 | | SET 1 | SET 2 | SET 3 | SET 4 | SET 5 | SET 6 | SET 7 | SET 8 | |
|---|---|---|---|---|---|---|---|---|---|---|
| Monday | Warm up | 7 | 9 | 7 | 7 | 10+ | — | — | — | Stretch |
| Tuesday | | | | | Rest | | | | | |
| Wednesday | Warm up | 8 | 10 | 8 | 8 | 11+ | — | — | — | Stretch |
| Thursday | | | | | Rest | | | | | |
| Friday | Warm up | 9 | 11 | 9 | 9 | 12+ | — | — | — | Stretch |
| Saturday | | | | | Rest | | | | | |
| Sunday | | | | | Rest | | | | | |

**Rest 60 seconds between each SET (longer if required)**

**Remember to warm up and stretch! See pages 140–165.**

*Note:* Rest and recovery are vital to the success of the programs and should be included as prescribed on the schedules.

## INTERMEDIATE 1

| Week 3 | | SET 1 | SET 2 | SET 3 | SET 4 | SET 5 | SET 6 | SET 7 | SET 8 | |
|---|---|---|---|---|---|---|---|---|---|---|
| Monday | Warm up | 9 | 12 | 9 | 9 | 14+ | — | — | — | Stretch |
| Tuesday | | | | | Rest | | | | | |
| Wednesday | Warm up | 10 | 13 | 10 | 10 | 16+ | — | — | — | Stretch |
| Thursday | | | | | Rest | | | | | |
| Friday | Warm up | 11 | 14 | 12 | 12 | 18+ | — | — | — | Stretch |
| Saturday | | | | | Rest | | | | | |
| Sunday | | | | | Rest | | | | | |

| Week 4 | | SET 1 | SET 2 | SET 3 | SET 4 | SET 5 | SET 6 | SET 7 | SET 8 | |
|---|---|---|---|---|---|---|---|---|---|---|
| Monday | Warm up | 12 | 15 | 12 | 12 | 18+ | — | — | — | Stretch |
| Tuesday | | | | | Rest | | | | | |
| Wednesday | Warm up | 14 | 16 | 14 | 14 | 19+ | — | — | — | Stretch |
| Thursday | | | | | Rest | | | | | |
| Friday | Warm up | 15 | 17 | 15 | 15 | 22+ | — | — | — | Stretch |
| Saturday | | | | | Rest | | | | | |
| Sunday | | | | | Rest | | | | | |

**Rest 60 seconds between each SET (longer if required)**

**Remember to warm up and stretch! See pages 140–165.**

*Note:* Rest and recovery are vital to the success of the programs and should be included as prescribed on the schedules.

## INTERMEDIATE 1

| Week 5 | | SET 1 | SET 2 | SET 3 | SET 4 | SET 5 | SET 6 | SET 7 | SET 8 | |
|---|---|---|---|---|---|---|---|---|---|---|
| Monday | Warm up | 16 | 20 | 16 | 15 | 26+ | — | — | — | Stretch |
| Tuesday | | | | | Rest | | | | | |
| Wednesday | Warm up | 10 | 10 | 16 | 16 | 10 | 10 | 31+ | — | Stretch |
| Thursday | | | | | Rest | | | | | |
| Friday | Warm up | 11 | 11 | 16 | 16 | 11 | 11 | 37+ | — | Stretch |
| Saturday | | | | | Rest | | | | | |
| Sunday | | | | | Rest | | | | | |

| Week 6 | | SET 1 | SET 2 | SET 3 | SET 4 | SET 5 | SET 6 | SET 7 | SET 8 | |
|---|---|---|---|---|---|---|---|---|---|---|
| Monday | Warm up | 12 | 12 | 22 | 22 | 40+ | — | — | — | Stretch |
| Tuesday | | | | | Rest | | | | | |
| Wednesday | Warm up | 14 | 14 | 18 | 18 | 14 | 14 | 44+ | — | Stretch |
| Thursday | | | | | Rest | | | | | |
| Friday | Warm up | 16 | 16 | 22 | 22 | 16 | 16 | 48+ | — | Stretch |
| Saturday | | | | | Rest | | | | | |
| Sunday | | | | | Rest | | | | | |

**Rest 60 seconds between each SET (longer if required)**

**Remember to warm up and stretch! See pages 140–165.**

*Note:* Rest and recovery are vital to the success of the programs and should be included as prescribed on the schedules.

## INTERMEDIATE 1

| Week 7 | | SET 1 | SET 2 | SET 3 | SET 4 | SET 5 | SET 6 | SET 7 | SET 8 | |
|---|---|---|---|---|---|---|---|---|---|---|
| Monday | Warm up | 14 | 20 | 19 | 20 | 50+ | — | — | — | Stretch |
| Tuesday | | | | | Rest | | | | | |
| Wednesday | Warm up | 18 | 18 | 20 | 20 | 16 | 16 | 16 | 55+ | Stretch |
| Thursday | | | | | Rest | | | | | |
| Friday | Warm up | 20 | 20 | 22 | 22 | 18 | 18 | 18 | 60+ | Stretch |
| Saturday | | | | | Rest | | | | | |
| Sunday | | | | | Rest | | | | | |
| | | Rest 60 seconds between each SET (longer if required) | | | | | | | | |
| | | Remember to warm up and stretch! See pages 140–165. | | | | | | | | |

*Note:* Rest and recovery are vital to the success of the programs and should be included as prescribed on the schedules.

## INTERMEDIATE 2

| Week 1 | | SET 1 | SET 2 | SET 3 | SET 4 | SET 5 | SET 6 | SET 7 | SET 8 | |
|---|---|---|---|---|---|---|---|---|---|---|
| Monday | Warm up | 6 | 8 | 6 | 6 | 7+ | — | — | — | Stretch |
| Tuesday | | | | | Rest | | | | | |
| Wednesday | Warm up | 8 | 10 | 8 | 8 | 9+ | — | — | — | Stretch |
| Thursday | | | | | Rest | | | | | |
| Friday | Warm up | 9 | 12 | 9 | 9 | 11+ | — | — | — | Stretch |
| Saturday | | | | | Rest | | | | | |
| Sunday | | | | | Rest | | | | | |

| Week 2 | | SET 1 | SET 2 | SET 3 | SET 4 | SET 5 | SET 6 | SET 7 | SET 8 | |
|---|---|---|---|---|---|---|---|---|---|---|
| Monday | Warm up | 9 | 11 | 9 | 9 | 12+ | — | — | — | Stretch |
| Tuesday | | | | | Rest | | | | | |
| Wednesday | Warm up | 10 | 12 | 10 | 10 | 13+ | — | — | — | Stretch |
| Thursday | | | | | Rest | | | | | |
| Friday | Warm up | 11 | 13 | 11 | 11 | 14+ | — | — | — | Stretch |
| Saturday | | | | | Rest | | | | | |
| Sunday | | | | | Rest | | | | | |

**Rest 60 seconds between each SET (longer if required)**

**Remember to warm up and stretch! See pages 140–165.**

*Note:* Rest and recovery are vital to the success of the programs and should be included as prescribed on the schedules.

## INTERMEDIATE 2

| Week 3 | | SET 1 | SET 2 | SET 3 | SET 4 | SET 5 | SET 6 | SET 7 | SET 8 | |
|---|---|---|---|---|---|---|---|---|---|---|
| Monday | Warm up | 11 | 14 | 11 | 11 | 16+ | — | — | — | Stretch |
| Tuesday | Rest | | | | | | | | | |
| Wednesday | Warm up | 12 | 15 | 12 | 12 | 18+ | — | — | — | Stretch |
| Thursday | Rest | | | | | | | | | |
| Friday | Warm up | 13 | 16 | 14 | 14 | 20+ | — | — | — | Stretch |
| Saturday | Rest | | | | | | | | | |
| Sunday | Rest | | | | | | | | | |

| Week 4 | | SET 1 | SET 2 | SET 3 | SET 4 | SET 5 | SET 6 | SET 7 | SET 8 | |
|---|---|---|---|---|---|---|---|---|---|---|
| Monday | Warm up | 14 | 17 | 14 | 14 | 20+ | — | — | — | Stretch |
| Tuesday | Rest | | | | | | | | | |
| Wednesday | Warm up | 16 | 18 | 16 | 16 | 21+ | — | — | — | Stretch |
| Thursday | Rest | | | | | | | | | |
| Friday | Warm up | 17 | 19 | 17 | 17 | 24+ | — | — | — | Stretch |
| Saturday | Rest | | | | | | | | | |
| Sunday | Rest | | | | | | | | | |

Rest 60 seconds between each SET (longer if required)

Remember to warm up and stretch! See pages 140–165.

## INTERMEDIATE 2

| Week 5 | | SET 1 | SET 2 | SET 3 | SET 4 | SET 5 | SET 6 | SET 7 | SET 8 | |
|---|---|---|---|---|---|---|---|---|---|---|
| Monday | Warm up | 18 | 22 | 18 | 18 | 28+ | — | — | — | Stretch |
| Tuesday | | | | | Rest | | | | | |
| Wednesday | Warm up | 12 | 12 | 18 | 18 | 12 | 12 | 33+ | — | Stretch |
| Thursday | | | | | Rest | | | | | |
| Friday | Warm up | 13 | 13 | 18 | 18 | 13 | 13 | 39+ | — | Stretch |
| Saturday | | | | | Rest | | | | | |
| Sunday | | | | | Rest | | | | | |
| **Week 6** | | SET 1 | SET 2 | SET 3 | SET 4 | SET 5 | SET 6 | SET 7 | SET 8 | |
| Monday | Warm up | 14 | 14 | 24 | 24 | 42+ | — | — | — | Stretch |
| Tuesday | | | | | Rest | | | | | |
| Wednesday | Warm up | 16 | 16 | 20 | 20 | 16 | 16 | 46+ | — | Stretch |
| Thursday | | | | | Rest | | | | | |
| Friday | Warm up | 18 | 18 | 24 | 24 | 18 | 18 | 50+ | — | Stretch |
| Saturday | | | | | Rest | | | | | |
| Sunday | | | | | Rest | | | | | |
| | | **Rest 60 seconds between each SET (longer if required)** | | | | | | | | |
| | | Remember to warm up and stretch! See pages 140–165. | | | | | | | | |

## INTERMEDIATE 2

| Week 7 | | SET 1 | SET 2 | SET 3 | SET 4 | SET 5 | SET 6 | SET 7 | SET 8 | |
|---|---|---|---|---|---|---|---|---|---|---|
| Monday | Warm up | 16 | 18 | 21 | 22 | 50+ | — | — | — | Stretch |
| Tuesday | | | | | Rest | | | | | |
| Wednesday | Warm up | 20 | 20 | 22 | 22 | 18 | 18 | 18 | 55+ | Stretch |
| Thursday | | | | | Rest | | | | | |
| Friday | Warm up | 22 | 22 | 24 | 24 | 20 | 20 | 20 | 60+ | Stretch |
| Saturday | | | | | Rest | | | | | |
| Sunday | | | | | Rest | | | | | |
| | Rest 60 seconds between each SET (longer if required) | | | | | | | | | |
| | Remember to warm up and stretch! See pages 140–165. | | | | | | | | | |

*Note:* Rest and recovery are vital to the success of the programs and should be included as prescribed on the schedules.

## ADVANCED 1

| Week 1 | | SET 1 | SET 2 | SET 3 | SET 4 | SET 5 | SET 6 | SET 7 | SET 8 | |
|---|---|---|---|---|---|---|---|---|---|---|
| Monday | Warm up | 11 | 13 | 8 | 8 | 10+ | — | — | — | Stretch |
| Tuesday | | | | | Rest | | | | | |
| Wednesday | Warm up | 11 | 13 | 9 | 9 | 13+ | — | — | — | Stretch |
| Thursday | | | | | Rest | | | | | |
| Friday | Warm up | 12 | 14 | 10 | 10 | 14+ | — | — | — | Stretch |
| Saturday | | | | | Rest | | | | | |
| Sunday | | | | | Rest | | | | | |
| **Week 2** | | SET 1 | SET 2 | SET 3 | SET 4 | SET 5 | SET 6 | SET 7 | SET 8 | |
| Monday | Warm up | 10 | 13 | 10 | 10 | 14+ | — | — | — | Stretch |
| Tuesday | | | | | Rest | | | | | |
| Wednesday | Warm up | 12 | 15 | 11 | 11 | 16+ | — | — | — | Stretch |
| Thursday | | | | | Rest | | | | | |
| Friday | Warm up | 14 | 17 | 12 | 12 | 18+ | — | — | — | Stretch |
| Saturday | | | | | Rest | | | | | |
| Sunday | | | | | Rest | | | | | |

**Rest 60 seconds between each SET (longer if required)**

**Remember to warm up and stretch! See pages 140–165.**

## ADVANCED 1

| Week 3 | | SET 1 | SET 2 | SET 3 | SET 4 | SET 5 | SET 6 | SET 7 | SET 8 | |
|---|---|---|---|---|---|---|---|---|---|---|
| Monday | Warm up | 12 | 15 | 10 | 10 | 17+ | — | — | — | Stretch |
| Tuesday | | | | | Rest | | | | | |
| Wednesday | Warm up | 14 | 17 | 12 | 12 | 19+ | — | — | — | Stretch |
| Thursday | | | | | Rest | | | | | |
| Friday | Warm up | 16 | 20 | 14 | 14 | 21+ | — | — | — | Stretch |
| Saturday | | | | | Rest | | | | | |
| Sunday | | | | | Rest | | | | | |

| Week 4 | | SET 1 | SET 2 | SET 3 | SET 4 | SET 5 | SET 6 | SET 7 | SET 8 | |
|---|---|---|---|---|---|---|---|---|---|---|
| Monday | Warm up | 13 | 17 | 13 | 13 | 19+ | — | — | — | Stretch |
| Tuesday | | | | | Rest | | | | | |
| Wednesday | Warm up | 19 | 20 | 14 | 14 | 24+ | — | — | — | Stretch |
| Thursday | | | | | Rest | | | | | |
| Friday | Warm up | 21 | 24 | 19 | 19 | 28+ | — | — | — | Stretch |
| Saturday | | | | | Rest | | | | | |
| Sunday | | | | | Rest | | | | | |

**Rest 60 seconds between each SET (longer if required)**

**Remember to warm up and stretch! See pages 140–165.**

## ADVANCED 1

| Week 5 | | SET 1 | SET 2 | SET 3 | SET 4 | SET 5 | SET 6 | SET 7 | SET 8 | |
|---|---|---|---|---|---|---|---|---|---|---|
| Monday | Warm up | 19 | 25 | 21 | 21 | 31+ | — | — | — | Stretch |
| Tuesday | | | | | Rest | | | | | |
| Wednesday | Warm up | 13 | 13 | 19 | 19 | 13 | 13 | 34+ | — | Stretch |
| Thursday | | | | | Rest | | | | | |
| Friday | Warm up | 13 | 13 | 20 | 20 | 13 | 13 | 36+ | — | Stretch |
| Saturday | | | | | Rest | | | | | |
| Sunday | | | | | Rest | | | | | |
| Week 6 | | SET 1 | SET 2 | SET 3 | SET 4 | SET 5 | SET 6 | SET 7 | SET 8 | |
| Monday | Warm up | 17 | 27 | 23 | 23 | 41+ | — | — | — | Stretch |
| Tuesday | | | | | Rest | | | | | |
| Wednesday | Warm up | 17 | 17 | 23 | 23 | 18 | 18 | 45+ | — | Stretch |
| Thursday | | | | | Rest | | | | | |
| Friday | Warm up | 19 | 19 | 25 | 25 | 20 | 20 | 49+ | — | Stretch |
| Saturday | | | | | Rest | | | | | |
| Sunday | | | | | Rest | | | | | |

**Rest 60 seconds between each SET (longer if required)**

**Remember to warm up and stretch! See pages 140–165.**

## ADVANCED 1

| Week 7 | | SET 1 | SET 2 | SET 3 | SET 4 | SET 5 | SET 6 | SET 7 | SET 8 | |
|---|---|---|---|---|---|---|---|---|---|---|
| Monday | Warm up | 19 | 31 | 25 | 25 | 50+ | — | — | — | Stretch |
| Tuesday | | | | | Rest | | | | | |
| Wednesday | Warm up | 19 | 19 | 23 | 23 | 19 | 19 | 22 | 55+ | Stretch |
| Thursday | | | | | Rest | | | | | |
| Friday | Warm up | 23 | 23 | 30 | 30 | 25 | 25 | 23 | 60+ | Stretch |
| Saturday | | | | | Rest | | | | | |
| Sunday | | | | | Rest | | | | | |

Rest 60 seconds between each SET (longer if required)

Remember to warm up and stretch! See pages 140–165.

## ADVANCED 2

| Week 1 | | SET 1 | SET 2 | SET 3 | SET 4 | SET 5 | SET 6 | SET 7 | SET 8 | |
|---|---|---|---|---|---|---|---|---|---|---|
| Monday | Warm up | 13 | 15 | 10 | 10 | 12+ | — | — | — | Stretch |
| Tuesday | | | | | Rest | | | | | |
| Wednesday | Warm up | 13 | 15 | 11 | 11 | 15+ | — | — | — | Stretch |
| Thursday | | | | | Rest | | | | | |
| Friday | Warm up | 14 | 16 | 12 | 12 | 16+ | — | — | — | Stretch |
| Saturday | | | | | Rest | | | | | |
| Sunday | | | | | Rest | | | | | |

| Week 2 | | SET 1 | SET 2 | SET 3 | SET 4 | SET 5 | SET 6 | SET 7 | SET 8 | |
|---|---|---|---|---|---|---|---|---|---|---|
| Monday | Warm up | 12 | 15 | 12 | 12 | 16+ | — | — | — | Stretch |
| Tuesday | | | | | Rest | | | | | |
| Wednesday | Warm up | 14 | 17 | 13 | 13 | 18+ | — | — | — | Stretch |
| Thursday | | | | | Rest | | | | | |
| Friday | Warm up | 16 | 19 | 14 | 14 | 20+ | — | — | — | Stretch |
| Saturday | | | | | Rest | | | | | |
| Sunday | | | | | Rest | | | | | |

**Rest 60 seconds between each SET (longer if required)**

**Remember to warm up and stretch! See pages 140–165.**

## ADVANCED 2

| Week 3 | | SET 1 | SET 2 | SET 3 | SET 4 | SET 5 | SET 6 | SET 7 | SET 8 | |
|---|---|---|---|---|---|---|---|---|---|---|
| Monday | Warm up | 12 | 15 | 10 | 10 | 19+ | — | — | — | Stretch |
| Tuesday | | | | | Rest | | | | | |
| Wednesday | Warm up | 14 | 17 | 12 | 12 | 21+ | — | — | — | Stretch |
| Thursday | | | | | Rest | | | | | |
| Friday | Warm up | 16 | 20 | 14 | 14 | 23+ | — | — | — | Stretch |
| Saturday | | | | | Rest | | | | | |
| Sunday | | | | | Rest | | | | | |

| Week 4 | | SET 1 | SET 2 | SET 3 | SET 4 | SET 5 | SET 6 | SET 7 | SET 8 | |
|---|---|---|---|---|---|---|---|---|---|---|
| Monday | Warm up | 15 | 19 | 15 | 15 | 21+ | — | — | — | Stretch |
| Tuesday | | | | | Rest | | | | | |
| Wednesday | Warm up | 21 | 23 | 16 | 16 | 26+ | — | — | — | Stretch |
| Thursday | | | | | Rest | | | | | |
| Friday | Warm up | 23 | 27 | 21 | 21 | 30+ | — | — | — | Stretch |
| Saturday | | | | | Rest | | | | | |
| Sunday | | | | | Rest | | | | | |

**Rest 60 seconds between each SET (longer if required)**

**Remember to warm up and stretch! See pages 140–165.**

*Note:* Rest and recovery are vital to the success of the programs and should be included as prescribed on the schedules.

## ADVANCED 2

| Week 5 | | SET 1 | SET 2 | SET 3 | SET 4 | SET 5 | SET 6 | SET 7 | SET 8 | |
|---|---|---|---|---|---|---|---|---|---|---|
| Monday | Warm up | 21 | 27 | 23 | 23 | 33+ | — | — | — | Stretch |
| Tuesday | | | | | Rest | | | | | |
| Wednesday | Warm up | 15 | 15 | 21 | 21 | 15 | 15 | 36+ | — | Stretch |
| Thursday | | | | | Rest | | | | | |
| Friday | Warm up | 15 | 15 | 22 | 22 | 15 | 15 | 38+ | — | Stretch |
| Saturday | | | | | Rest | | | | | |
| Sunday | | | | | Rest | | | | | |
| Week 6 | | SET 1 | SET 2 | SET 3 | SET 4 | SET 5 | SET 6 | SET 7 | SET 8 | |
| Monday | Warm up | 18 | 28 | 24 | 24 | 42+ | — | — | — | Stretch |
| Tuesday | | | | | Rest | | | | | |
| Wednesday | Warm up | 18 | 18 | 24 | 24 | 19 | 19 | 46+ | — | Stretch |
| Thursday | | | | | Rest | | | | | |
| Friday | Warm up | 20 | 20 | 26 | 26 | 21 | 21 | 50+ | — | Stretch |
| Saturday | | | | | Rest | | | | | |
| Sunday | | | | | Rest | | | | | |

**Rest 60 seconds between each SET (longer if required)**

**Remember to warm up and stretch! See pages 140–165.**

*Note:* Rest and recovery are vital to the success of the programs and should be included as prescribed on the schedules.

## ADVANCED 2

| Week 7 | | SET 1 | SET 2 | SET 3 | SET 4 | SET 5 | SET 6 | SET 7 | SET 8 | |
|---|---|---|---|---|---|---|---|---|---|---|
| Monday | Warm up | 20 | 32 | 26 | 26 | 50+ | — | — | — | Stretch |
| Tuesday | | | | | Rest | | | | | |
| Wednesday | Warm up | 20 | 20 | 24 | 24 | 20 | 20 | 23 | 55+ | Stretch |
| Thursday | | | | | Rest | | | | | |
| Friday | Warm up | 24 | 24 | 31 | 31 | 26 | 26 | 24 | 60+ | Stretch |
| Saturday | | | | | Rest | | | | | |
| Sunday | | | | | Rest | | | | | |
| | | Rest 60 seconds between each SET (longer if required) | | | | | | | | |
| | | Remember to warm up and stretch! See pages 140–165. | | | | | | | | |

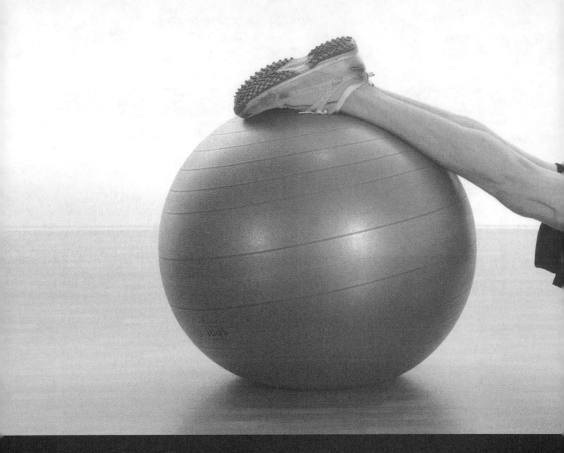

# MAINTENANCE

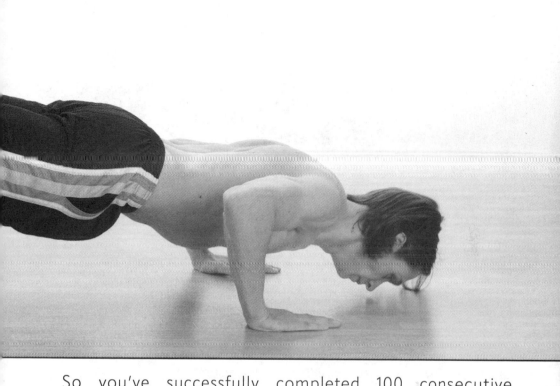

So you've successfully completed 100 consecutive push-ups, and naturally you're feeling pretty pleased with yourself. Nothing wrong with that; you've worked very hard to achieve the goal! I would also hazard a guess that you have noticed some pretty significant changes to your body—your chest will be more defined, shoulders broader, and arms toned and hard. Your abdominal muscles should be firmer, your posture more upright, and your energy level higher.

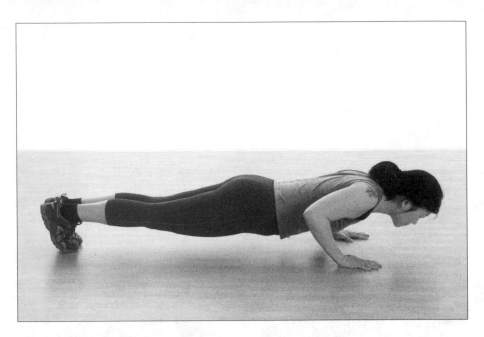

The amazing thing is that you're just getting started. Think about what you'll be able to accomplish with regular, long-term exercise if you can achieve so much in as little as seven weeks of doing push-ups.

Some people will be happy to have conquered the challenge and be content to find some other program to follow. This is completely fine, as variety of exercise will keep individuals motivated for longer periods. Why not look around for a basic weight-training plan or a new aerobic activity to try out? Train for your first 5K, take up yoga, or join a local swimming club. The possibilities are endless, but hopefully, you now have the confidence and base fitness to tackle almost anything.

Others, not content with doing 100 push-ups, will strive to reach 150, 200, or even more. For you people, I recommend restarting one of the main training plans and following along as you did the first time around. The only difference should be to increase the maximum set at the end of each workout. Not only will this help to maintain your current fitness level, but it will maximize your strength gains and take you to new limits. The sky is the limit if you keep challenging yourself!

Finally, if you're looking for more variety and are keen to hone in on your muscle development, Part 3 of the book contains a wide selection of advanced push-up variations that will really provide a challenge. For example, choose wide push-ups to target chest development or one-arm push-ups to develop strong forearms and chiseled triceps.

The main thing is to keep exercise fun and change up the routine every couple of months. Typically, after six to eight weeks, your body will have made all the adaptations it is going to make from that particular plan. You'll need to "shock the system" to keep making improvements and strength gains. Also, it would be wise to take a week or so of complete rest every two to three months—there's nothing like a short break to recharge yourself both mentally and physically.


Good luck!

# PART 3:

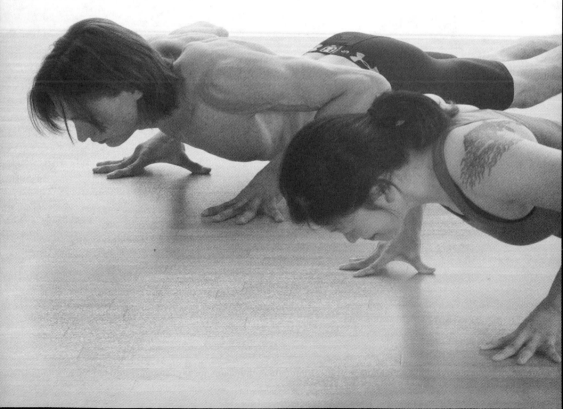

# BEYOND 100 PUSH-UPS

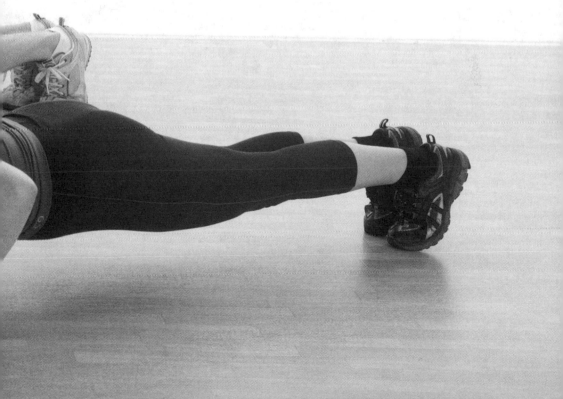

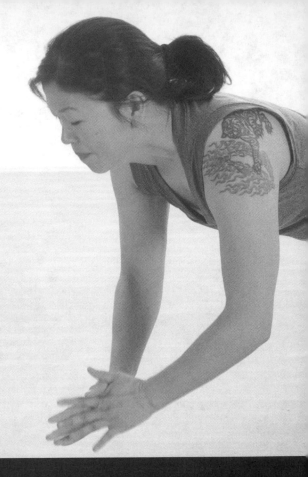

# CHALLENGING YOURSELF

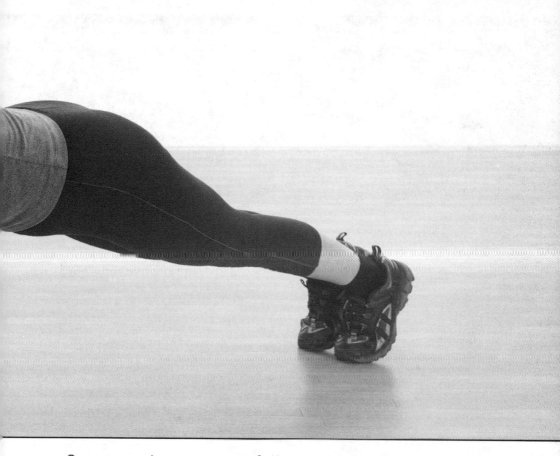

Once you have successfully completed 100 consecutive push-ups, either during the initial test (yes, it has been done!) or after following one of the six progressive training programs, you may have caught the push-ups bug and feel inclined to challenge yourself further. If you do fancy a little variety, there are many more challenging push-up exercises that will provide you with a more intense workout and target different parts of the body.

On July 25, 2000, Sergeant Paul Dean of the Royal Marines achieved a record 116 push-ups in one minute at the Marine training base in Lympstone, U.K. That same year on October 26, Yvan de Weber of Switzerland did 93 one-arm push-ups in one minute. De Weber's record was beaten by Jeremiah Gould of the U.S. on November 10, 2007, with a whopping 135 one-arm push-ups in one minute.

Of course, you may simply just wish to maintain your newfound strength and fitness, in which case this section of the book is not really applicable to you. Just in case you missed it, a basic maintenance routine is discussed on page 96.

Step-by-step instructions for some of the most popular challenging push-up variations are detailed on the following pages. Take some time to read through the instructions and study the diagrams to discover which areas of the body the specific exercise will target.

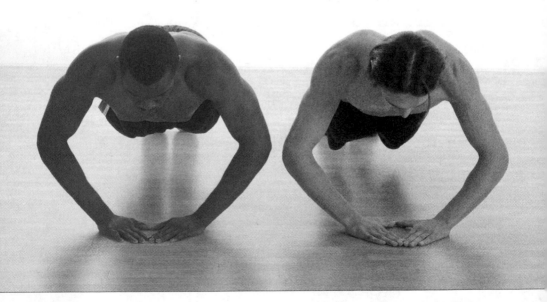

Once you've found one you like the sound of, consider performing an initial test as per page 60 before starting one of the six progressive training programs—Beginner 1 or 2, Intermediate 1 or 2, Advanced 1 or 2. Unlike the traditional push-up, you'll need some basic equipment to perform a few of these more challenging moves, including a stability/yoga ball, a medicine ball, a stool/low chair, and a BOSU.

There really is no limit to the strength and stability gains you can make by performing regular push-ups, and as with most forms of exercise, consistency is the key to success. If you're a little bored with the traditional push-up, however, these challenging moves will help keep workouts interesting and definitely make it easier to stay motivated.

# Wide push-up

*This variation in hand position changes the focus on the muscles being exercised and puts more emphasis on the chest rather than the arms and shoulders.*

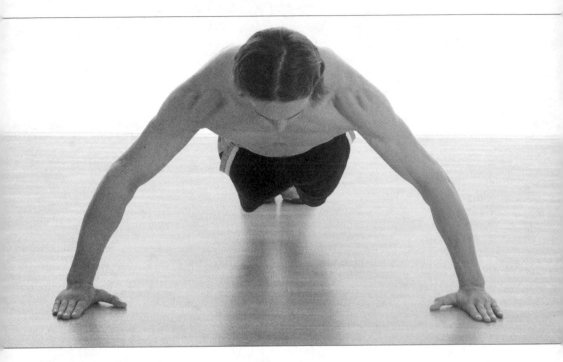

**STARTING POSITION:** Assume standard push-up position but place your hands on the floor about 6 to 9 inches wider than shoulder-width apart. Make sure your elbows don't flare out past your hands. Maintain a straight line from your shoulders to your feet by keeping your abs tight. Do not raise your butt in the air or allow your back to sag to the ground.

**1** Breathe in as you lower your torso to the ground, stopping when your elbows form a 90-degree angle and your chest is an inch or two from the ground.

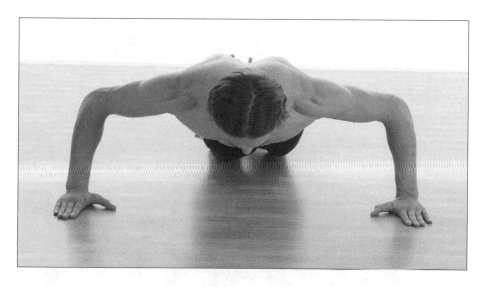

**2** Breathe out as you push yourself up using your arms. Think of raising yourself by attempting to push the ground away from you. The power for the push will predominantly come from your triceps, shoulders, and chest.

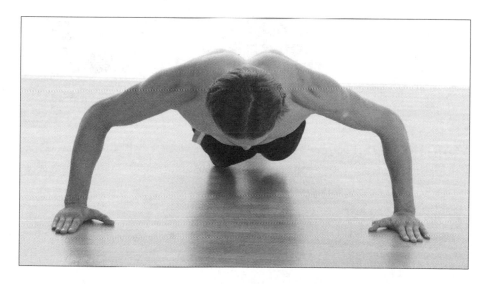

# Narrow push-up

*This variation in hand position concentrates on the triceps more than the chest and shoulders.*

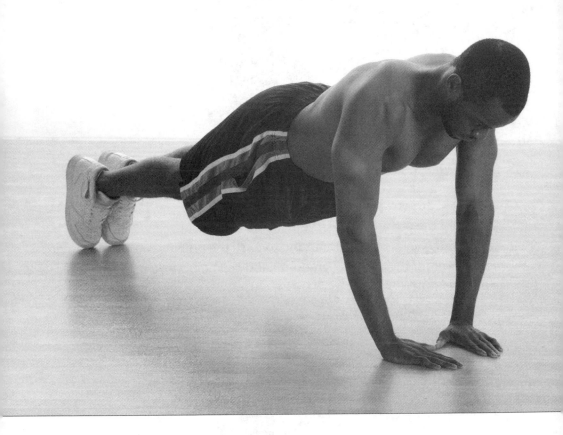

**STARTING POSITION:** Assume standard push-up position but place your hands directly under your chest, a couple of inches away from each other. To help with balance, consider spreading your legs slightly.

**1** Breathe in as you lower your torso to the ground, stopping when your elbows form a 90-degree angle and your chest is an inch or two from your hands. Keep your elbows close to your body.

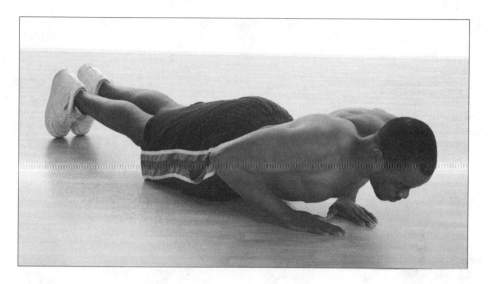

**2** Breathe out as you push yourself up using your arms. Think of raising yourself by attempting to push the ground away from you. The power for the push will predominantly come from your triceps, shoulders, and chest.

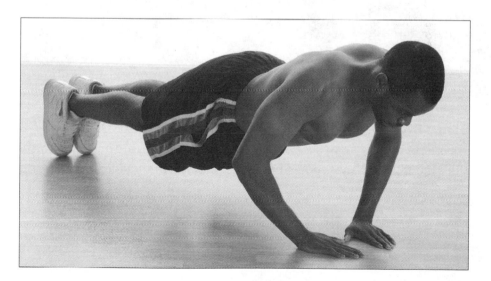

# Fingertip push-up

*This variation strengthens the chest, wrists, and forearms.*

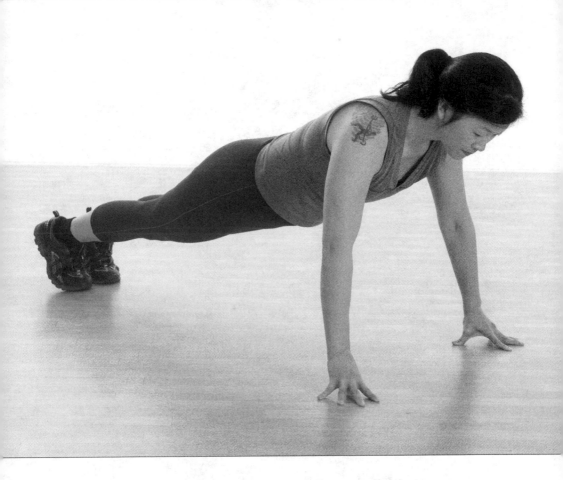

**STARTING POSITION:** Assume standard push-up position but make a "bear claw" with your hands so that only your fingertips are in contact with the ground. Your hands should be slightly wider than shoulder-width apart.

**1** Breathe in as you lower your torso to the ground until your chest is about an inch or two from the ground. Keep your elbows close to your body.

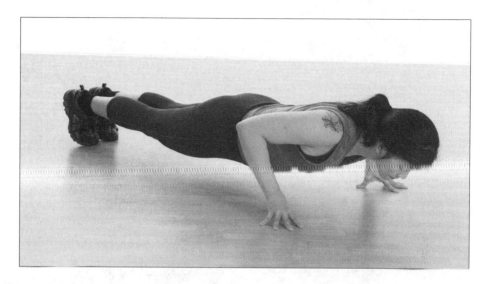

**2** Breathe out as you push yourself up using your arms. Think of raising yourself by attempting to push the ground away from you. The power for the push will predominantly come from your shoulders and chest.

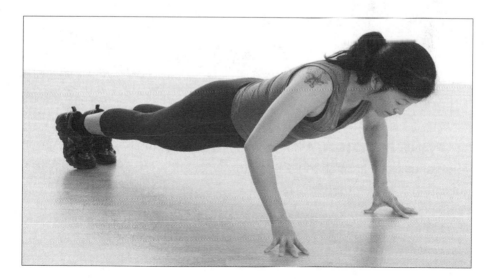

# Diamond push-up

*Much like the narrow push-up, this variation in hand position will concentrate on the triceps more than the chest and shoulders.*

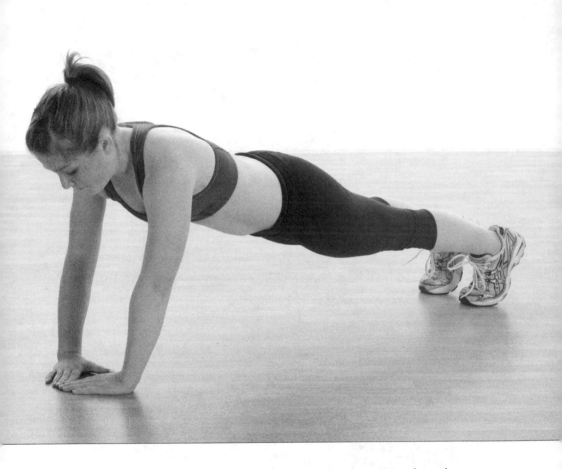

**STARTING POSITION:** Assume standard push-up position but place your hands close enough together to form a diamond shape with your index fingers and thumbs.

**1** Breathe in as you lower your torso to the ground until your chest is as close to the diamond as possible. Keep your elbows close to your body.

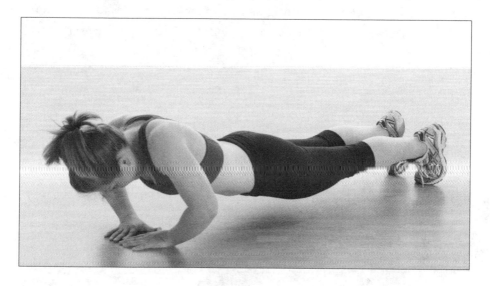

**2** Breathe out as you push yourself up using your arms.

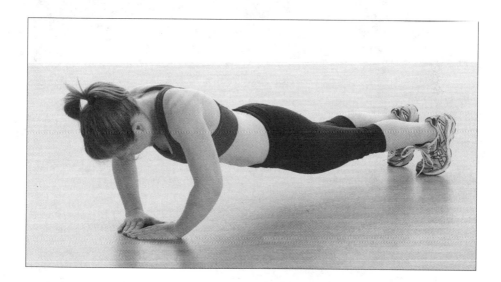

# Knuckle push-up

*A surprising number of people experience wrist discomfort as they perform regular push-ups, but by closing your hands and making fists, your body weight ends up on your knuckles instead of your palms, thus avoiding the wrist extension motion.*

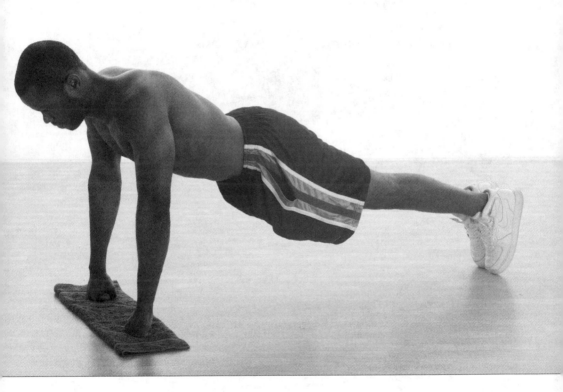

**STARTING POSITION:** Assume standard push-up position but place the knuckles of your fists (instead of your palms) on the floor perpendicular to the body.

*Note:* Please be sure to do this type of push-up on a padded mat, plush carpet, or even better, a folded towel.

**1** Breathe in as you lower your torso to the ground, stopping when your elbows form a 90-degree angle and your chest is inches from your hands. Keep your elbows close to your body.

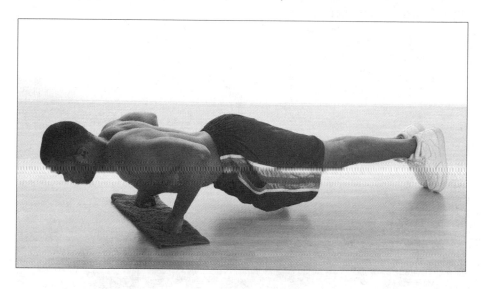

**2** Breathe out as you push yourself up using your arms. Think of raising yourself by attempting to push the ground away from you. The power for the push will predominantly come from your shoulders and chest.

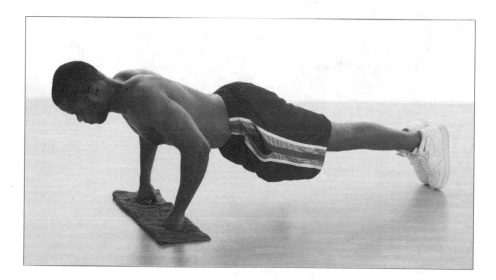

# Clapping push-up

*This explosive plyometric movement further develops the shoulders and chest, with an ancillary benefit to the triceps.*

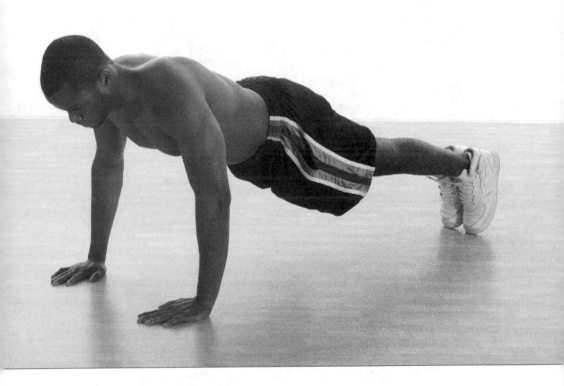

**STARTING POSITION:** Assume standard push-up position. To help with balance, consider spreading your legs slightly.

**1** Lower your torso to the ground, stopping when your elbows form a 90-degree angle and your chest is an inch or two from your hands.

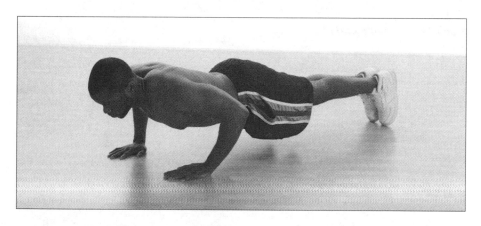

**2** Without pausing, immediately push your body back up as fast as possible. As your hands leave the ground, rapidly clap them together and place them back on the ground in starting position.

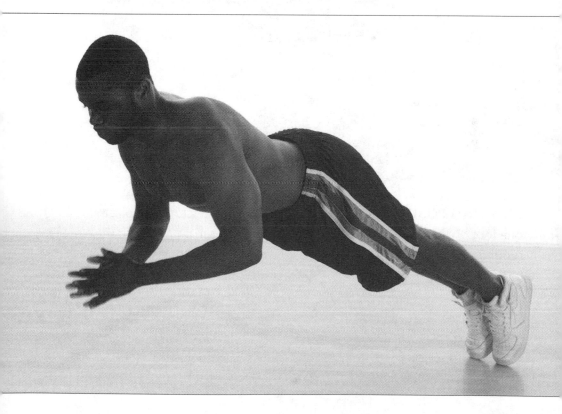

# One-leg push-up

*This push-up adds an element of balance, core stability, and increased strength requirement to the workout.*

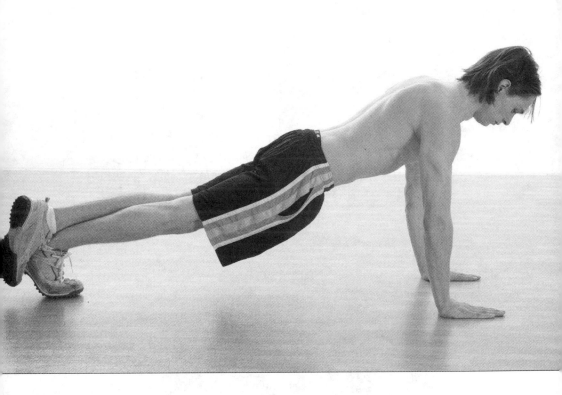

**STARTING POSITION:** Assume standard push-up position but place one foot on top of the other so only the lower foot is in contact with the ground.

**1** Breathe in as you lower your torso to the ground, stopping when your elbows form a 90-degree angle and your chest is an inch or two from your hands. Keep your elbows close to your body.

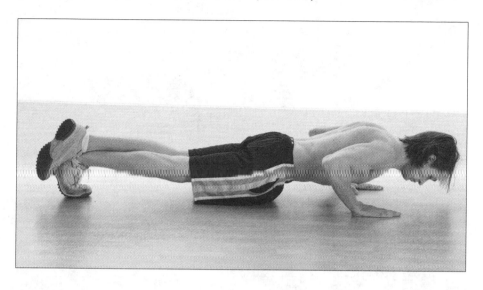

**2** Breathe out as you push yourself up using your arms. Think of raising yourself by attempting to push the ground away from you. The power for the push will predominantly come from your shoulders and chest.

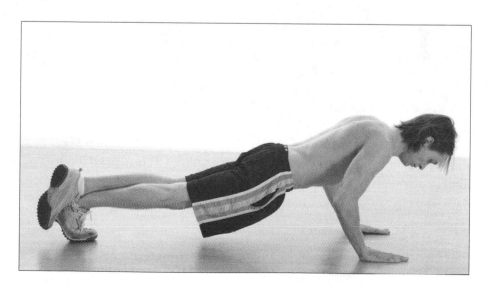

# One-arm push-up

*This variation strengthens the chest, triceps, and forearms.*

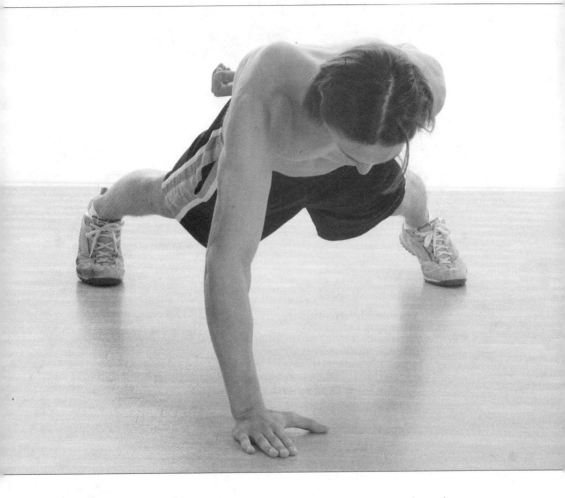

**STARTING POSITION:** Assume standard push-up position but place your feet slightly wider than shoulder-width apart. Lift one hand (your weaker one) and rest it on the small of your back.

**1** To maintain balance, turn your torso slightly away from the pushing arm. Breathe in as you lower your angled torso to the ground until your chin is a few inches above the floor.

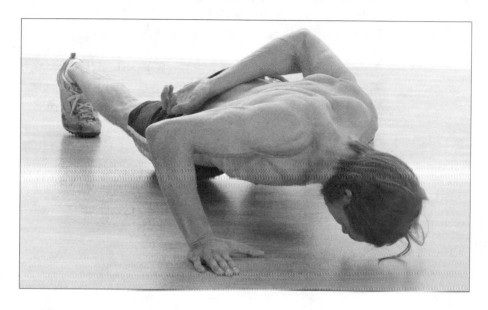

**2** Breathe out as you push yourself up from the floor, keeping your back straight. Stop just before you lock out your elbow at the top of the movement.

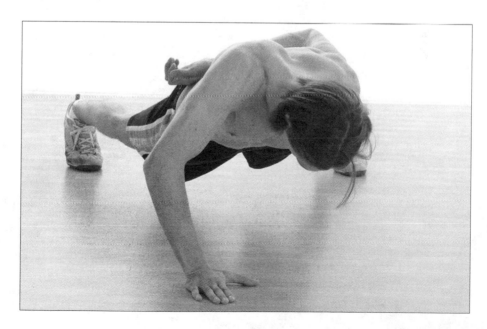

# Hands on stability ball push-up

*This push-up activates all upper-body and core muscle groups for balance and stabilization.*

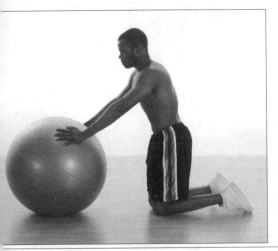

**STARTING POSITION:** Kneel behind the ball and place your hands shoulder-width apart on the sides of the ball. Move your feet back and lean forward so that your chest is directly over the ball and you are supported on your toes.

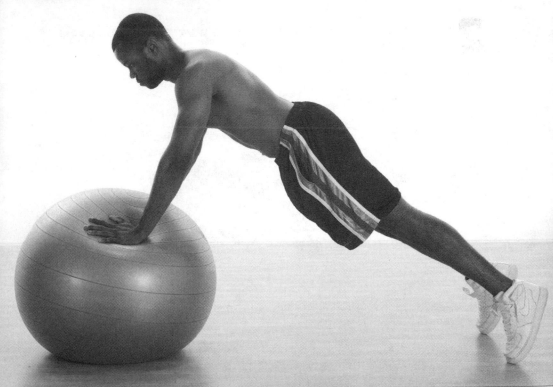

**1** Beathe in and bend your arms to lower your chest to the ball until your elbows form a 90-degree angle. Maintain a strong core and do not allow your hips to relax and drop. Hold for one to two seconds at the bottom.

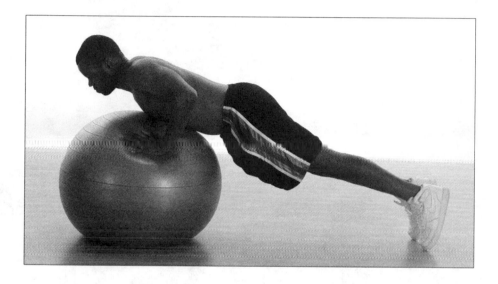

**2** Breathe out and extend your arms to bring your upper body back to starting position.

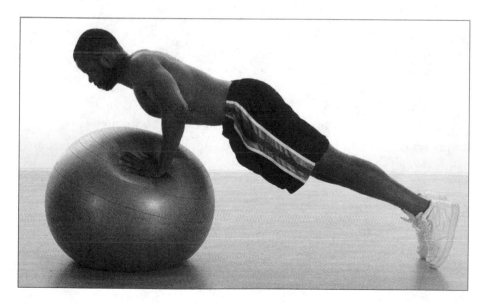

# Feet on stability ball push-up

*This variation strengthens the chest, back, and triceps and helps flatten the abdominal muscles.*

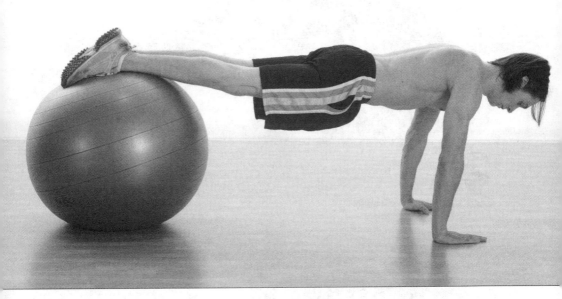

**STARTING POSITION:** Lie face-down on the ball with your arms supporting you in push-up position. Roll forward until your pelvis and thighs are off the ball and your feet are positioned on top of the ball. Your hands should be directly beneath your shoulders.

**1** Breathe in as you lower yourself by bending your arms until your elbows form a 90-degree angle. Use your core muscles to stabilize yourself.

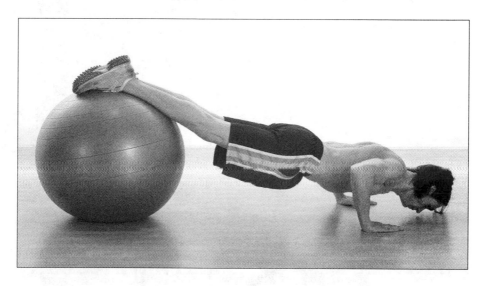

**2** Pause for one to two seconds at the bottom before breathing out and using your arms to push yourself up to starting position.

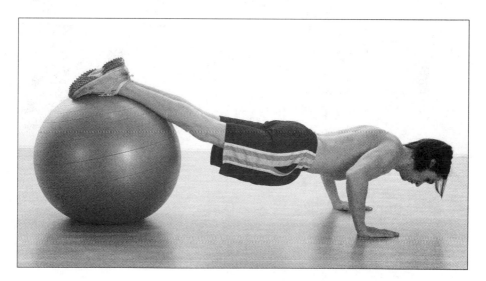

# Hands on medicine ball push-up

*This push-up adds an element of balance, core stability, and increased strength requirement to the workout.*

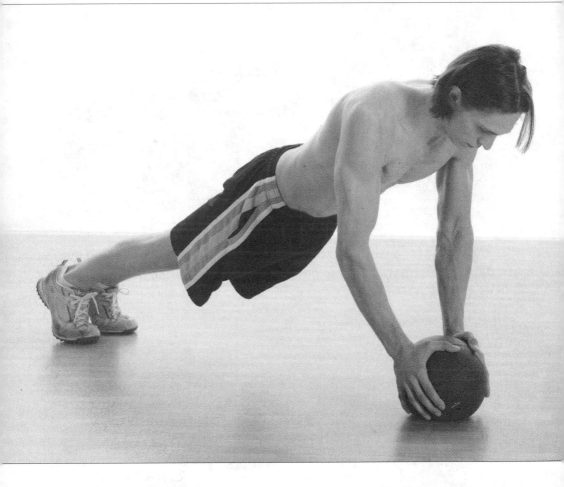

**STARTING POSITION:** Place a medicine ball in front of you. Assume a prone position and place your hands at 3 o'clock and 9 o'clock on the ball. You may keep your feet shoulder-width apart for better balance.

**1** Breathe in and bend your elbows to lower yourself in a controlled manner. Maintain a rigid core as your chest moves toward the top of the ball.

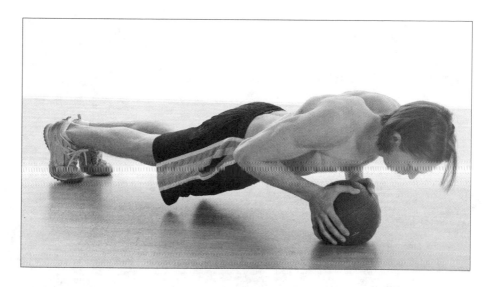

**2** Hold for one to two seconds before breathing out, extending your arms and pushing your body back to starting position. Focus on maintaining balance during both phases.

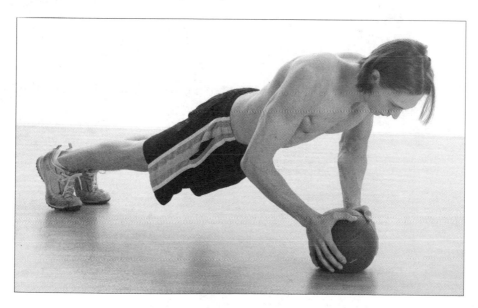

# Elevated feet push-up

*This push-up increases the demand on your upper chest and arms.*

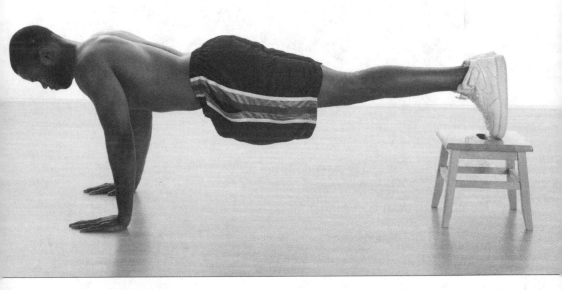

**STARTING POSITION:** Assume standard push-up position but place the balls of both feet on a well-supported stool or low chair.

**1** Breathe in as you lower your torso until your chest is just a fraction of an inch off the floor.

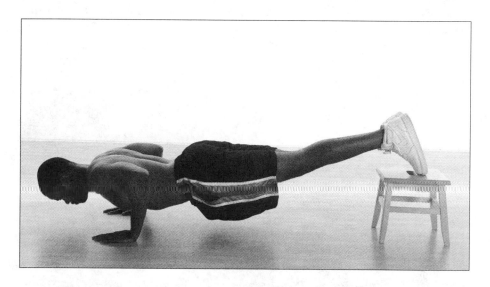

**2** Hold for one to two seconds before breathing out and extending your arms, pushing your body back to starting position.

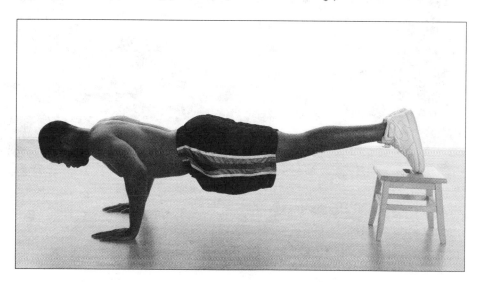

# BOSU dome push-up

*This push-up adds an element of balance, core stability, and increased strength requirement to the workout.*

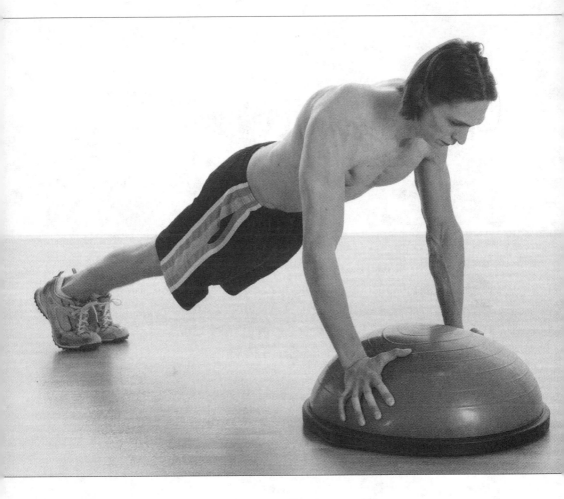

**STARTING POSITION:** Place your hands on the sides of the BOSU dome and assume standard push-up position.

**1** Breathe in and bend your arms to lower your body down as far as you can manage—ideally to within an inch or two of the BOSU. Maintain a straight line from head to ankle.

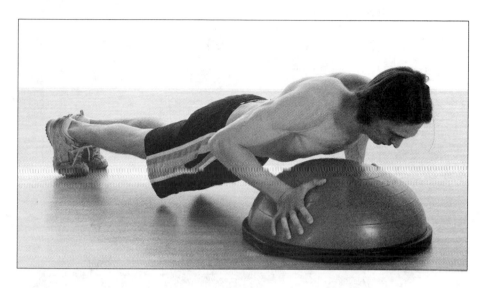

**2** Breathe out and push back to starting position using your chest, upper back and arm muscles. Maintain balance by keeping a strong core.

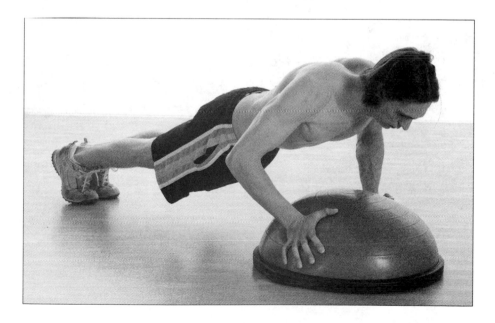

# BOSU platform push-up

*This push-up adds an element of balance, core stability, and increased strength requirement to the workout.*

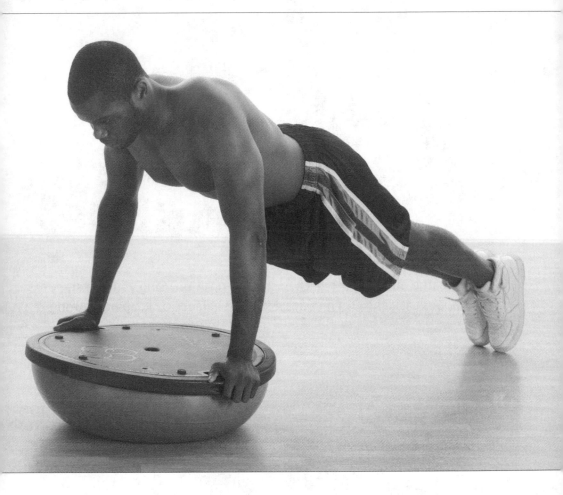

**STARTING POSITION:** Grasp the handles on either side of the BOSU platform and assume standard push-up position.

**1** Breathe in and bend your arms to lower your body down as far as you can manage—ideally to within an inch or two of the BOSU. Maintain a straight line from head to ankle.

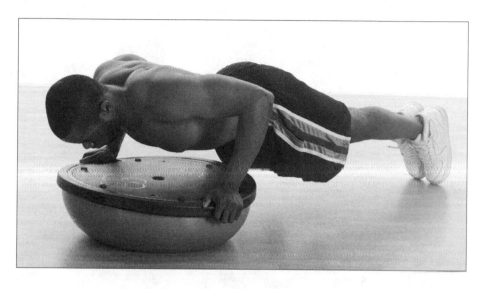

**2** Breathe out and push back to starting position using your chest, upper back, and arm muscles. Maintain balance by keeping a strong core.

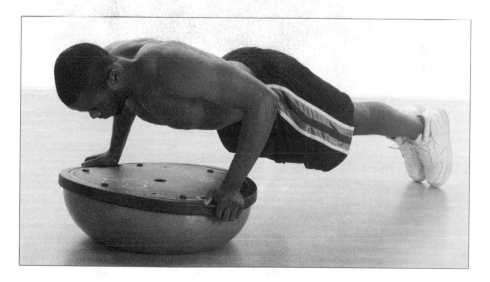

# Switch push-up

*This push-up increases the demand on the shoulders and triceps, and also introduces an aerobic element to the workout.*

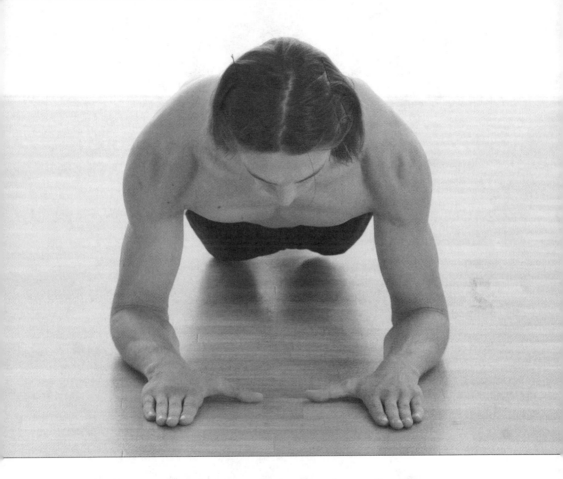

**STARTING POSITION:** Assume a standard plank position on your elbows and toes, with your body in a straight line from head to ankles. Maintain this position by engaging your core and making sure you don't allow your hips to sag.

**1** Breathe out and push yourself up on your right hand.

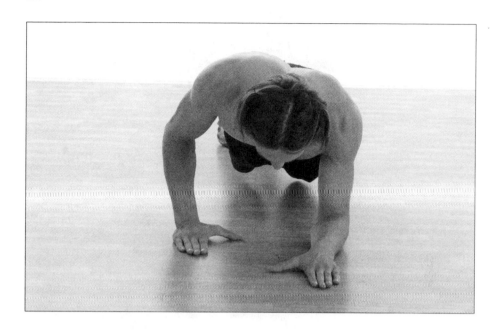

**2** Now switch and push up on your left hand. You should now be in the regular push-up starting position.

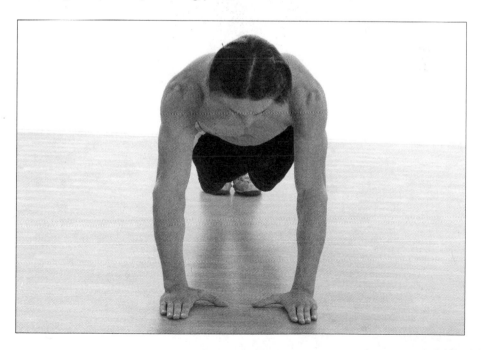

**3** Lower yourself to your left elbow.

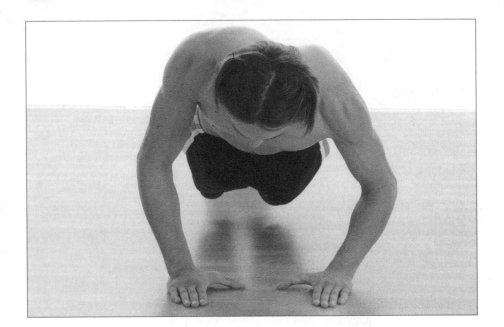

**7 WEEKS TO 100 PUSH-UPS**

**4** 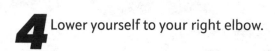 Lower yourself to your right elbow.

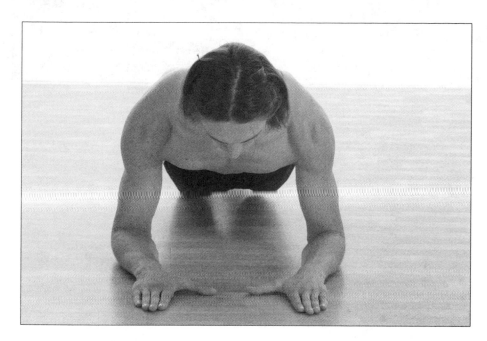

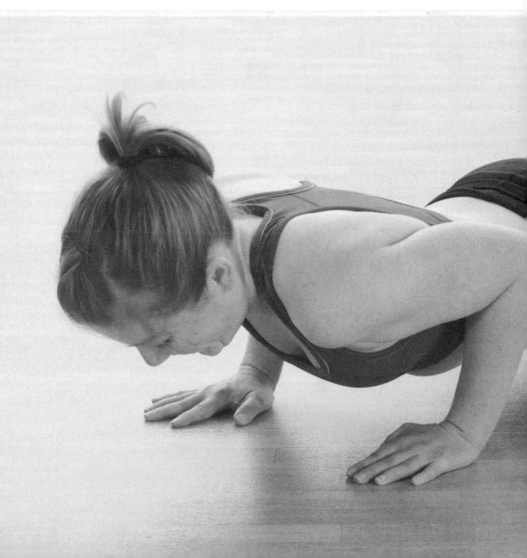

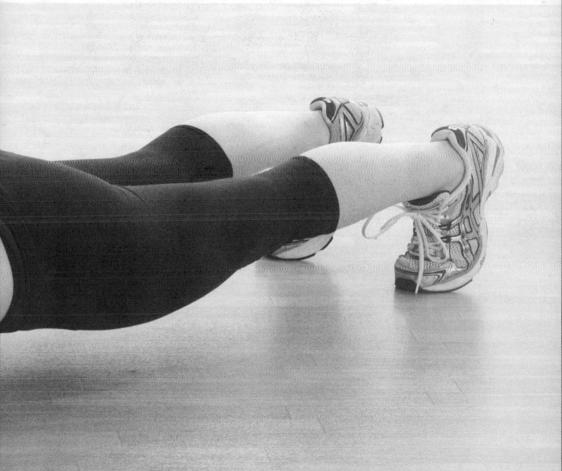

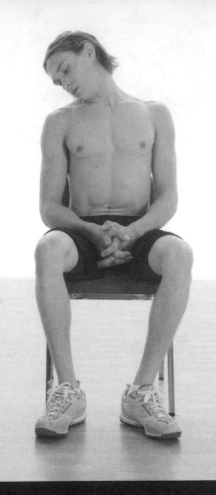 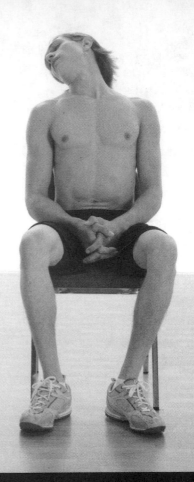

*7 WEEKS TO 100 PUSH-UPS*

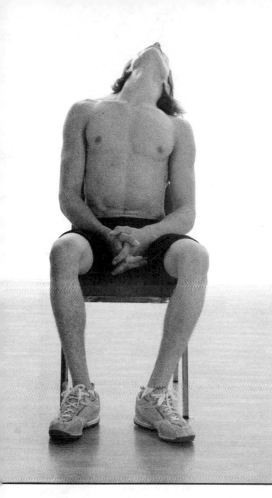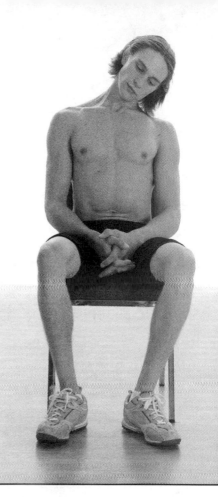

To maximize the gains from any workout, a thorough warm-up is crucial. For this reason, it's important to take the time to raise your body temperature and both your heart and breathing rates. An effective warm-up will also mobilize the joints and alert the nerve-to-muscle pathways to prime your body for the activity it's about to undertake.

Warming up doesn't have to take a long time, but it pays to be thorough and spend a solid 10 minutes or so to prepare for the push-ups you're about to undertake. Remember, a thorough warm-up will improve your subsequent performance and reduce the risk of injury.

For the sake of simplicity, I've broken down the warm-up routine into the following stages:

- **GENTLE MOBILITY** Easy movements that allow your joints to move freely.

- **PULSE RAISER** Gentle, progressive, aerobic activity that start the process of raising your heart rate.

- **SPECIFIC MOBILITY** Dynamic, exercise-specific movements that aid joint mobility.

- **FINAL PULSE RAISER** The last stage of preparing your heart rate and body temperature for exercise.

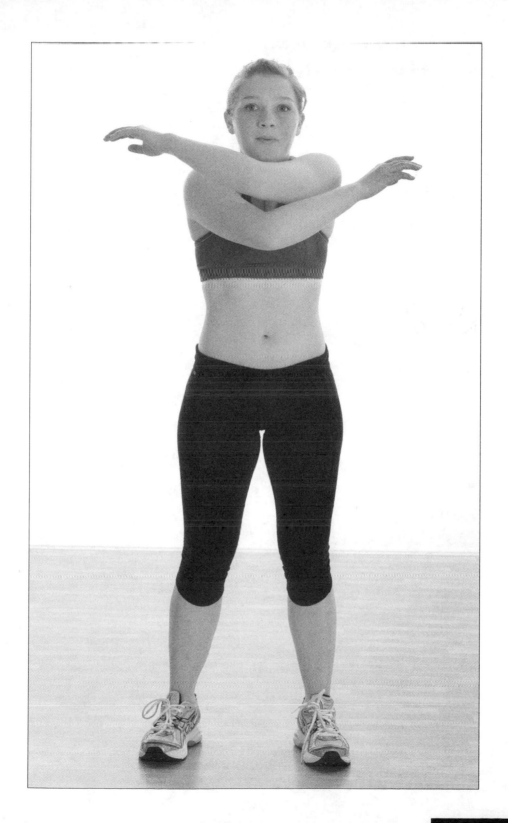

# Gentle Mobility

*The purpose of these gentle movements is to mobilize the joints. Perform each of them while stationary, and try to do each movement 7 or 8 times.*

## Neck

**STARTING POSITION:** Sit tall on a bench or sturdy chair.

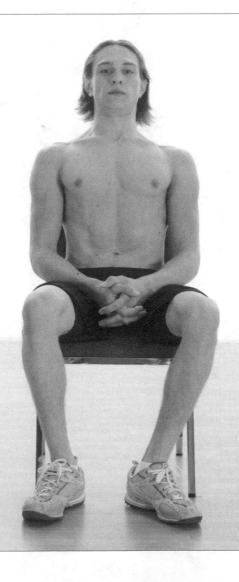

**1** Slide your head directly to the left and then the right.

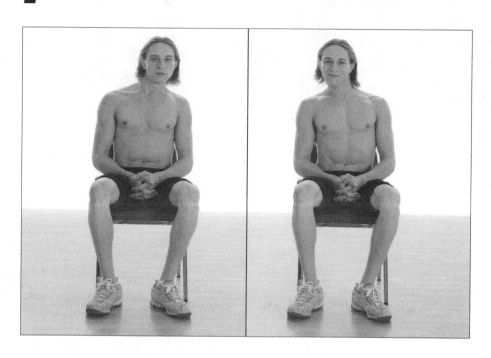

**2** Next, gently move your head backward, then drop your chin to your chest.

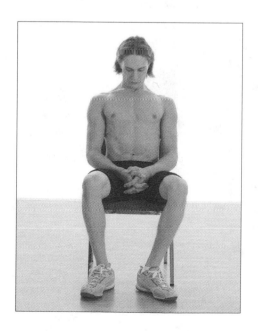

**3** Next, turn your head to the left and then the right.

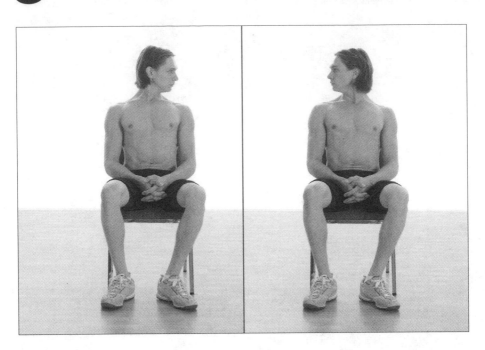

**4** Finally, facing forward, rotate your head clockwise. When you return to the starting point, rotate your head counterclockwise.

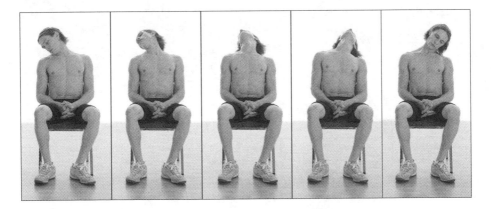

# *Shoulders*

**STARTING POSITION:** Stand tall.

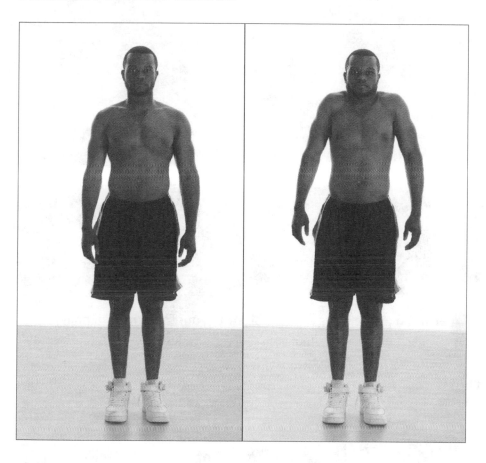

**1** Shrug your shoulders up to your ears, and then roll them backward and down.

## STARTING POSITION:
Stand with your feet hip-width apart.

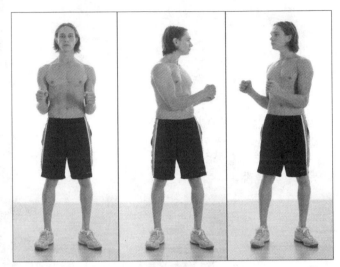

**1** Position your elbows at your waist with your forearms extending forward and slowly rotate your torso to the left and right. Make sure to keep your hips centered.

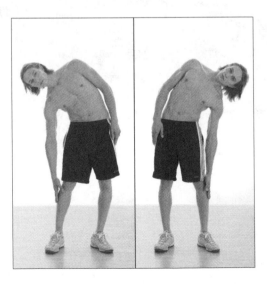

**2** Now drop your hands to your sides and slide each hand in turn down the outside of your thigh, bending your trunk to each side alternately.

# Pulse Raiser

*The aim of the initial pulse raiser is to raise your body temperature and elevate your heart rate. Start by walking briskly in place, gradually building up to a gentle running action over the course of 2 to 4 minutes. Try to maintain good posture and think about your balance at all times. It may help to focus on a spot on the wall in front of you, rather than keep your head in a lowered position.*

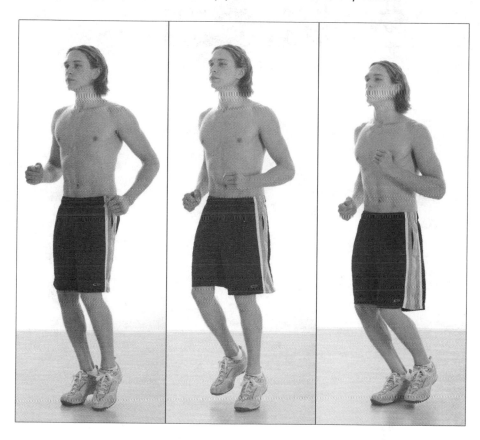

# Specific Mobility

*The purpose of these movements is to further mobilize the joints. Perform the following dynamic movements to prepare your upper body for the upcoming push-ups workout.*

## Arms and shoulders

**STARTING POSITION:** Stand tall.

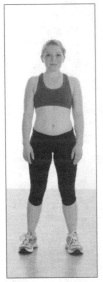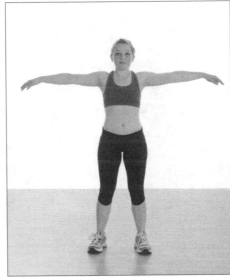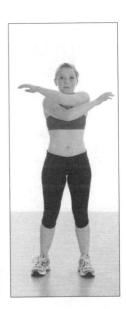

**1** Hold your arms out to your sides at shoulder level.

**2** Bring them together and cross them in front of your body. Return to starting position and repeat 6 to 8 times.

# *Arm circles*

**STARTING POSITION:** Stand tall.

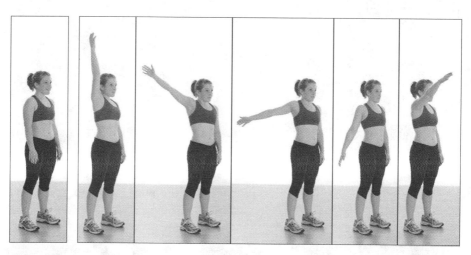

**1** Extend your right arm straight up past your ear and then rotate it backward in a large circle. Repeat 6 to 8 times, and then switch arms.

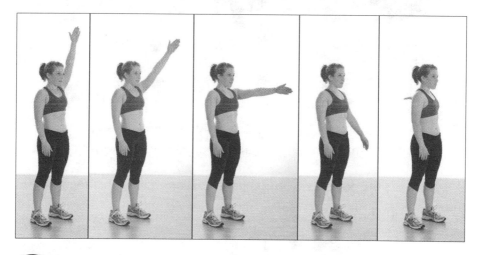

**2** Rotate your left arm forward 6 to 8 times, followed by the same exercise with your right arm.

**STARTING POSITION:** Stand with your feet hip-distance apart and hold your arms up by your ears.

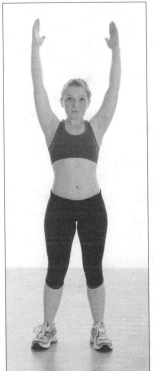 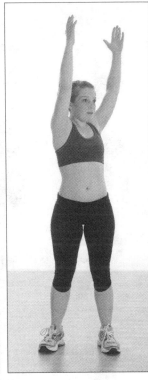 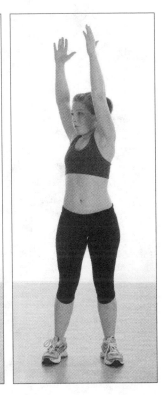

**1** Keeping your hips facing forward, gently twist your torso to the left, leading with your arms and allowing your head to follow your spine.

**2** Twist to the opposite side. Repeat 6 to 8 times in each direction.

# Final Pulse Raiser

The aim of the final pulse raiser is to further raise your body temperature and heart rate. Start by running gently in place, gradually picking up the pace over the course of 2 to 4 minutes. Try to maintain good posture and think about your balance at all times. It may help to focus on a spot on the wall in front of you, rather than keep your head in a lowered position.

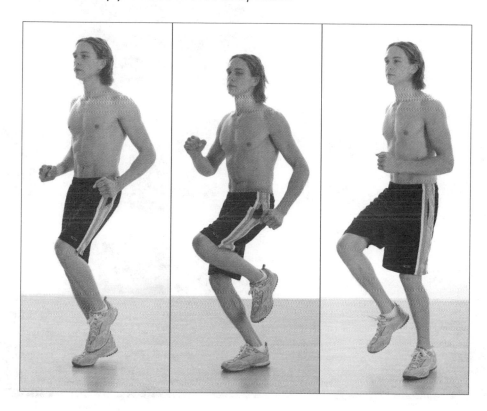

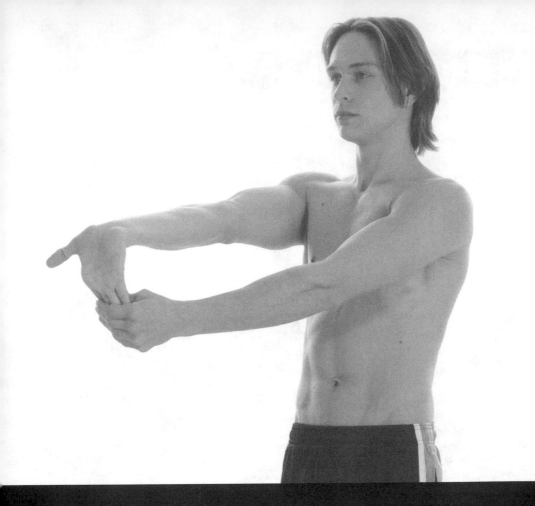

# STRETCHES

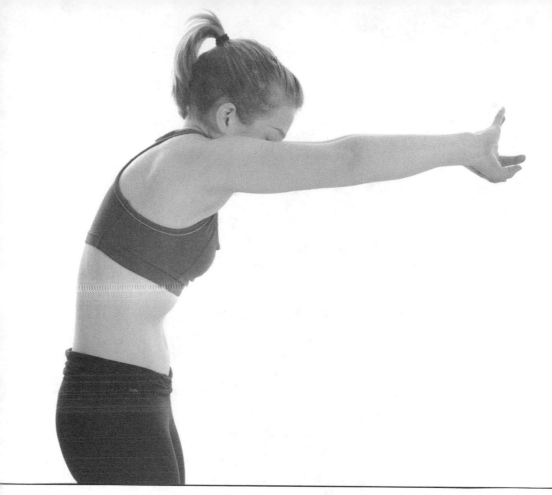

Stretching can be defined as the process of elongating muscles and connective tissues and is crucial to the success of any exercise regime. The benefits of post-exercise stretching far outweigh those of pre-exercise stretching but, remember, it's also very important to warm up thoroughly before performing any form of exercise.

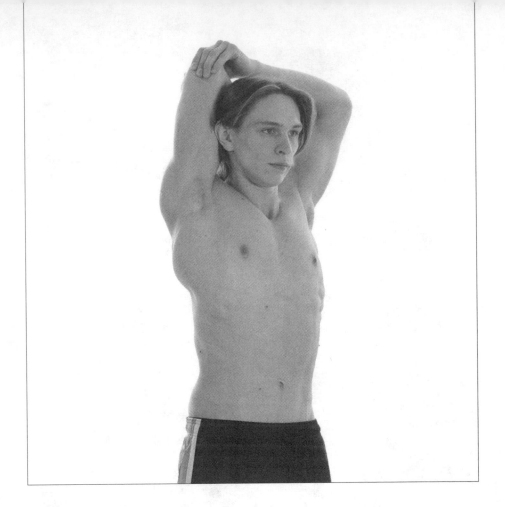

Stretching immediately post-exercise when the muscles are still warm will yield the best results. In addition, there is less chance of injury and the muscles and connective tissues are more likely to respond favorably at this time.

Stretching, for many people, is the most relaxing part of a workout and has the added benefits of returning your muscles to their resting length and improving flexibility over time. Improving flexibility will increase the range of movement around a joint or a group of joints, which in turn helps to strengthen the joint as well as increase the flow of blood into the muscles around it. In contrast, flexibility will quickly diminish over time when the connective tissues are not stretched or exercised.

The practice of stretching after exercise will:

- Help your breathing and heart rate gradually return to their normal states.

- Help prepare your muscles for the next exercise session. The next session could be the next day or in a few days' time.

- Help remove waste products such as lactic acid from your muscles, which can build up during strenuous activity.

- Help reduce the risk of muscle strain during exercise.

- Help reduce muscle tension and soreness post-exercise.

- Help promote development of general body awareness.

To maximize the stretching phase of the workout, ensure you stretch each major muscle group that you have used during the push-ups routine. Stretch each of the following muscle groups for the respective amount of time. Repeat if so desired.

*Important:* Stretching is beneficial but only if performed correctly. To avoid serious injury, please take note of the following guidelines:

- Perform each stretch slowly and deliberately.

- Focus on the muscle you're trying to stretch and try to lengthen it.

- Hold the stretch for the stated period of time. Longer is not necessarily better.

- Breathe normally and relax while holding the stretch.

- Don't stretch past the point of discomfort. Stretching should not be painful.

-  Don't perform "bouncy" stretching. Always hold and relax.

- If a muscle group is tight, stretch it in stages. Stretch as far as you can, relax it, and stretch again.

- Remember to stretch both sides of the body.

- Move slowly out of the stretch before moving on to the next muscle group.

- Stretching with excessive force is likely to add to muscle damage and delay the recovery process.

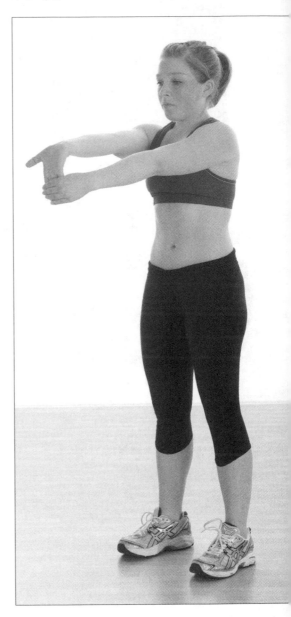

# Neck

Stand tall and move your right ear to your right shoulder, stretching out the left side of your neck.

To increase the stretch, take your hand over your head and gently pull the head further to the side.

Hold for 10–15 seconds, then swap sides and repeat.

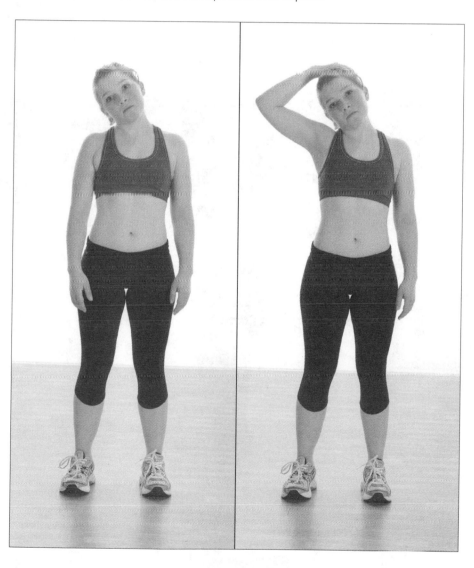

# Chest

Stand tall and clasp your hands together behind your back, palms pointing upward.

Gently pull your arms away from your back, keeping your arms as straight as possible and your shoulders down.

Hold for 10–15 seconds, lower, and repeat.

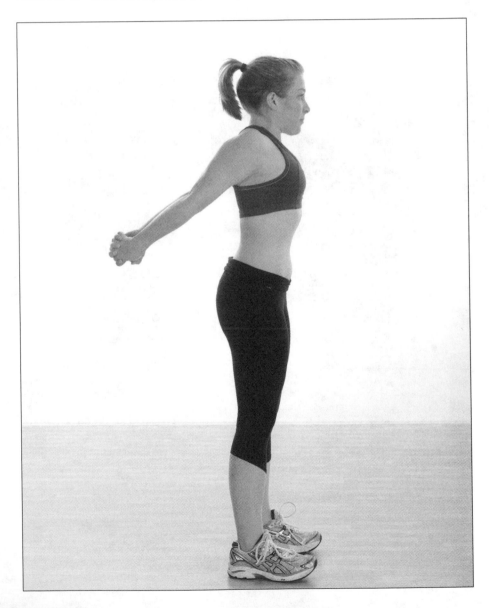

# Shoulders

Stand tall with your feet hip-distance apart. Take your right arm across your body, grasping it just above the elbow with the crook of your left arm. Gently pull your arm into your chest, taking care not to hunch your shoulders

Hold for 10–15 seconds, then swap sides and repeat.

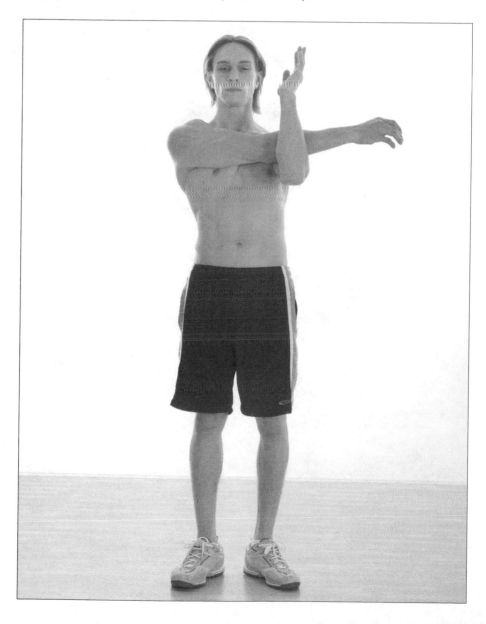

# Back and shoulders

Stand with your feet hip-width apart and knees slightly bent. Interlace your fingers together in front of your body. Push away through your shoulders and upper back, rounding your back into a C shape.

Hold for 10–15 seconds, relax ,and repeat.

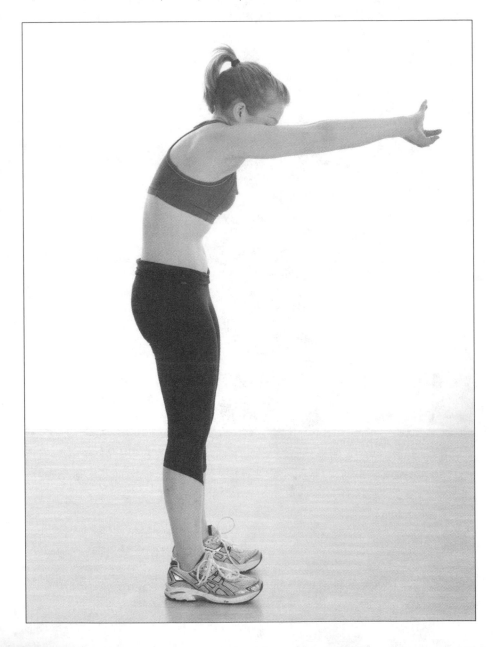

# Back

Lie face down on the floor and raise yourself up onto your forearms. Position your elbows directly below your shoulders, with your forearms extended forward and palms flat and in full contact with the floor. Press your hipbones into the floor and allow your back to extend. Be sure to keep your eyes looking forward—not up or down.

Hold for 10–15 seconds.

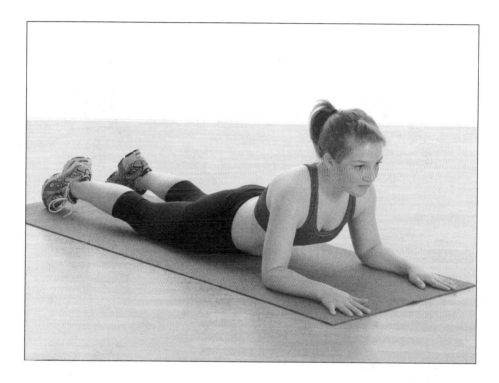

# Forearm and wrist

Stand with your feet hip-width apart and extend both arms out in front of you. Turn your left hand upward and use your right hand to gently pull your fingers toward your body. Feel a stretch along the underside of your arm and wrist.

Hold for 10 seconds, swap arms, and repeat.

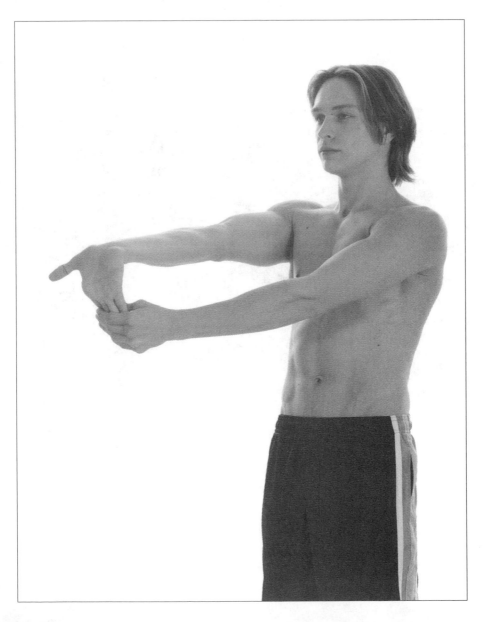

**7 WEEKS TO 100 PUSH-UPS**

# Triceps

Stand with your feet hip-width apart and extend your right arm above your head. Bending the elbow, drop your forearm behind your head. Gently push the elbow back with your left hand.

Hold for 10–15 seconds, swap arms, and repeat.

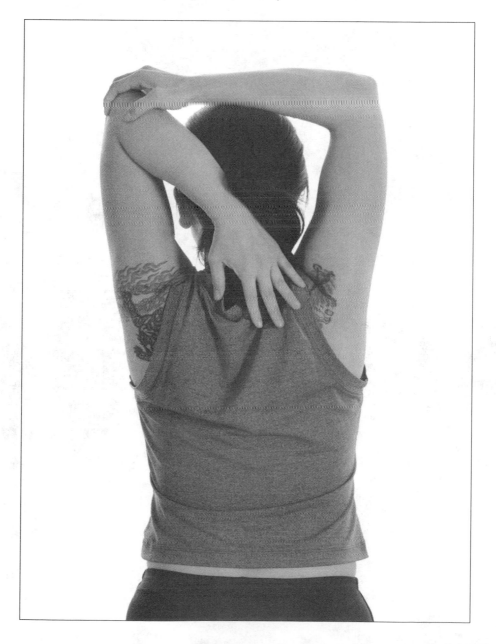

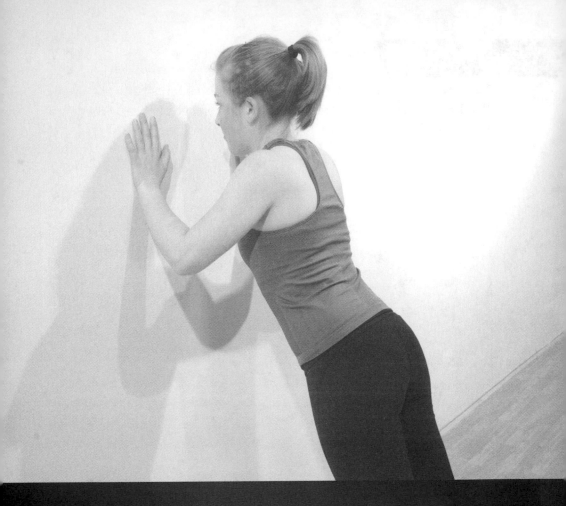

# PRELIMINARY PROGRAM

**7 WEEKS TO 100 PUSH-UPS**

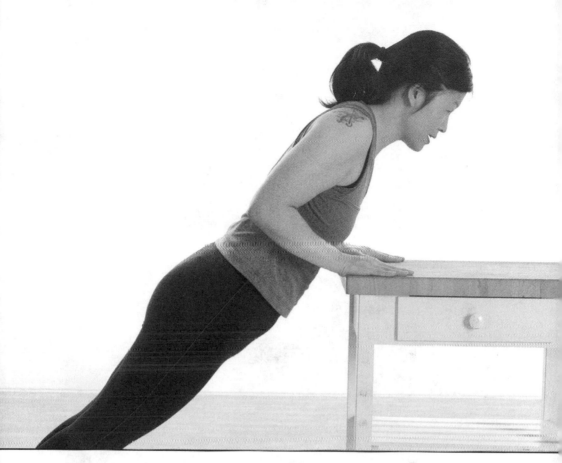

So you've tried the "good-form" push-ups but can only manage one or two before exhaustion sets in. Hey, you may even have struggled to do one single push-up. Don't be too discouraged—there are several options that will still enable you to follow the *7 Weeks to 100 Push-Ups* plan.

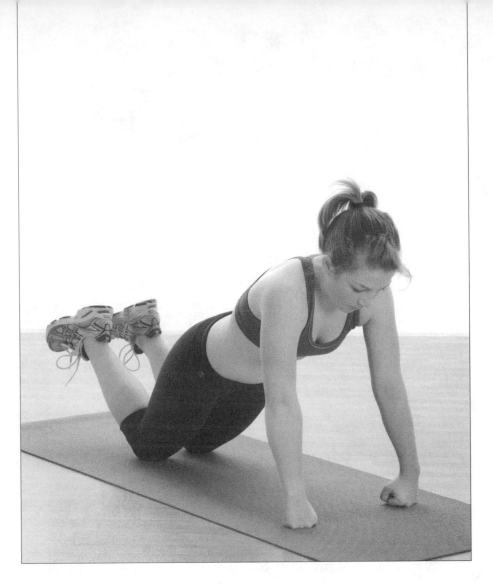

Remember, the main aim of the 100 push-ups program is to improve your strength, fitness, and general health. It really doesn't matter which style of push-up you perform as long as you continue to make progress and keep challenging yourself.

# Four-Week Program

Prepare yourself for the *7 Weeks to 100 Push-Ups* plan with this four-week preliminary program, which utilizes less challenging yet very effective exercises. Exercising on a Monday, Wednesday, and Friday works well and allows you to use the weekend for rest and recovery before moving on to the next stage of the program. Feel free to juggle the plan around to meet your busy schedule, but please make sure you rest in between workout days. You can chart your progress with a Preliminary Program Push-Ups Log starting on 194.

In **WEEK 1** of the preliminary program, you'll be performing "wall" push-ups—five sets of varying reps, each with 60 seconds of recovery time. **WEEK 2** is a similar format but you'll test your new strength and move up to "table" push-ups. You'll step it up once again for **WEEK 3** by performing the more challenging "chair" push-ups, before finally dispensing with the props and doing unassisted knee push-ups during **WEEK 4**.

Once you've worked your way through this preliminary program, you should be ready to tackle the *7 Weeks to 100 Push-Ups* plan. However, if you struggled at all with any of the weeks, I recommend you go back to repeat the week in question before moving on to the next week.

*Note:* Please remember to familiarize yourself with the exercises, paying close attention to the instructions and photos on pages 172–181, before starting this four-week preliminary program.

# PRELIMINARY WEEK 1: WALL PUSH-UPS

|  |  | SET 1 | SET 2 | SET 3 | SET 4 | SET 5 | SET 6 | SET 7 | SET 8 |  |
|---|---|---|---|---|---|---|---|---|---|---|
| Monday | Warm up | 5 | 8 | 5 | 5 | 10 | — | — | — | Stretch |
| Tuesday | Rest |  |  |  |  |  |  |  |  |  |
| Wednesday | Warm up | 6 | 10 | 6 | 6 | 12 | — | — | — | Stretch |
| Thursday | Rest |  |  |  |  |  |  |  |  |  |
| Friday | Warm up | 7 | 12 | 7 | 7 | 15 | — | — | — | Stretch |
| Saturday | Rest |  |  |  |  |  |  |  |  |  |
| Sunday | Rest |  |  |  |  |  |  |  |  |  |

# PRELIMINARY WEEK 2: TABLE PUSH-UPS

|  |  | SET 1 | SET 2 | SET 3 | SET 4 | SET 5 | SET 6 | SET 7 | SET 8 |  |
|---|---|---|---|---|---|---|---|---|---|---|
| Monday | Warm up | 5 | 8 | 5 | 5 | 10 | — | — | — | Stretch |
| Tuesday | Rest |  |  |  |  |  |  |  |  |  |
| Wednesday | Warm up | 6 | 10 | 6 | 6 | 12 | — | — | — | Stretch |
| Thursday | Rest |  |  |  |  |  |  |  |  |  |
| Friday | Warm up | 7 | 12 | 7 | 7 | 15 | — | — | — | Stretch |
| Saturday | Rest |  |  |  |  |  |  |  |  |  |
| Sunday | Rest |  |  |  |  |  |  |  |  |  |

Rest 60 seconds between each SET (longer if required)

Remember to warm up and stretch! See pages 140–165.

# PRELIMINARY WEEK 3: CHAIR PUSH-UPS

|  |  | SET 1 | SET 2 | SET 3 | SET 4 | SET 5 | SET 6 | SET 7 | SET 8 |  |
|---|---|---|---|---|---|---|---|---|---|---|
| Monday | Warm up | 5 | 8 | 5 | 5 | 10 | — | — | — | Stretch |
| Tuesday | | | | | Rest | | | | | |
| Wednesday | Warm up | 6 | 10 | 6 | 6 | 12 | — | — | — | Stretch |
| Thursday | | | | | Rest | | | | | |
| Friday | Warm up | 7 | 12 | 7 | 7 | 15 | — | — | — | Stretch |
| Saturday | | | | | Rest | | | | | |
| Sunday | | | | | Rest | | | | | |

# PRELIMINARY WEEK 4: KNEE PUSH-UPS

|  |  | SET 1 | SET 2 | SET 3 | SET 4 | SET 5 | SET 6 | SET 7 | SET 8 |  |
|---|---|---|---|---|---|---|---|---|---|---|
| Monday | Warm up | 5 | 8 | 5 | 5 | 10 | — | — | — | Stretch |
| Tuesday | | | | | Rest | | | | | |
| Wednesday | Warm up | 6 | 10 | 6 | 6 | 12 | — | — | — | Stretch |
| Thursday | | | | | Rest | | | | | |
| Friday | Warm up | 7 | 12 | 7 | 7 | 15 | — | — | — | Stretch |
| Saturday | | | | | Rest | | | | | |
| Sunday | | | | | Rest | | | | | |

**Rest 60 seconds between each SET (longer if required)**

**Remember to warm up and stretch! See pages 140–165.**

# Wall push-up

The "wall" push-up dramatically reduces the pressure on the arms, upper back, and abs. The closer you stand to the wall, the easier it is to perform, but remember, it's still important to be aware of your body alignment as you perform this push-up.

**STARTING POSITION:** Stand approximately 2 to 2.5 feet away from a large, empty wall with your arms held at shoulder height in front of you. Place your hands on the wall.

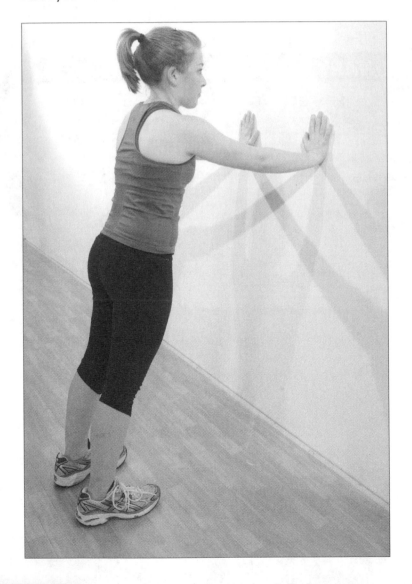

**1** Keeping your feet firmly fixed to the ground, lean your body forward so that your elbows flex and your chest comes within inches of the wall. Try not to flare your elbows to the sides.

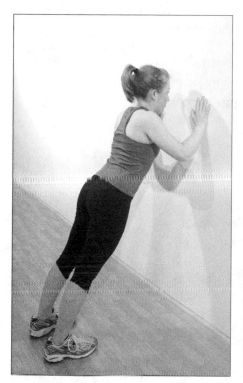
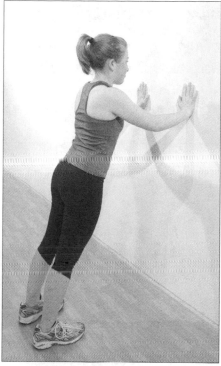

**2** Using your hands, push your body back into a standing position. The movement should be smooth and controlled.

# Counter/table push-up

Slightly more challenging than the wall push-up but still offering several degrees of assistance, the counter or table push-up is a very effective exercise that will target your upper back muscles and engage your triceps.

**STARTING POSITION:** Stand approximately 2.5 to 3 feet away from a waist-high countertop or sturdy table. Keeping your feet firmly on the ground, hold the front edge of the countertop or table with your hands, which should be slightly wider than shoulder-width apart.

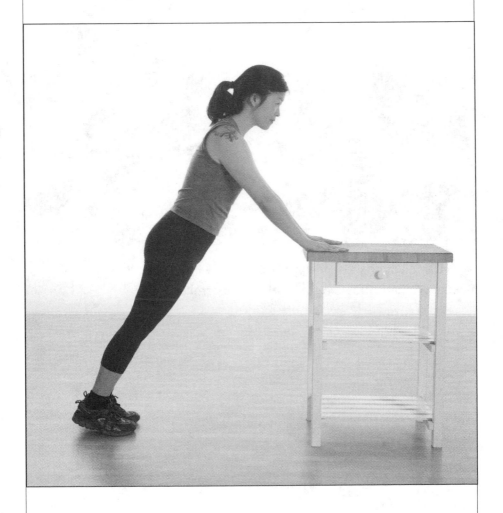

**1** Slowly lower yourself by flexing your elbows so that your chest comes within a few inches of the edge of the counter or table. Try not to flare your elbows to the sides.

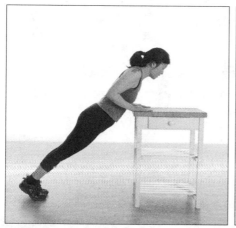 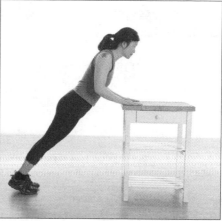

**2** Using your hands, push yourself back to starting position while focusing on maintaining a straight body position from head to ankle. The movement should be smooth and controlled.

# Bench/chair push-up

*For the next degree of difficulty, swap the table for a low bench or chair to support your arms while you perform regular push-ups. This type of push-up allows you to really concentrate on the push-up motion—all without the strain of the traditional version.*

**STARTING POSITION:** Stand approximately 3 to 3.5 feet away from a low bench or sturdy chair. Reach forward and grab the sides of the chair or front of the bench, keeping the balls of your feet in contact with the ground.

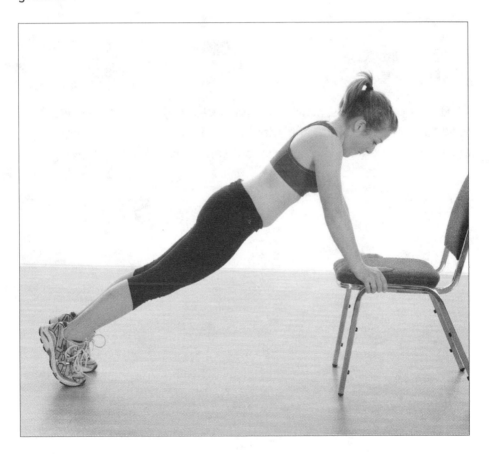

**1** Slowly lower yourself by flexing your elbows so that your chest comes within a few inches of the edge of the chair or bench. Try not to flare your elbows to the sides.

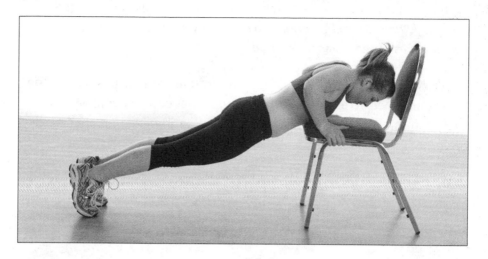

**2** Using your hands, push yourself back to starting position while focusing on maintaining a straight body position from head to ankle. The movement should be smooth and controlled.

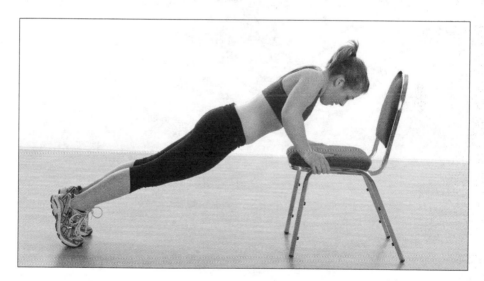

# Knee push-up

*To reduce the lifting load by about 50 percent, you can modify the traditional push-up position by doing the exercise on your knees. Keeping a straight line from neck to torso is still important, so please pay attention to correct body alignment as you perform this push-up.*

**STARTING POSITION:** Assume a comfortable kneeling position on the floor. It may help to place a towel or exercise mat under your knees for extra comfort. Slowly walk your arms forward until your hands are directly underneath your shoulders.

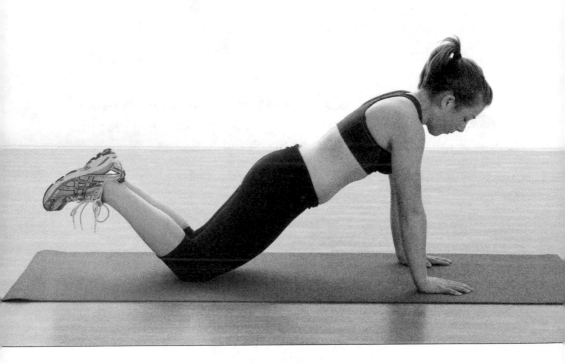

**1** Lower yourself by flexing your elbows so that your chest comes within a few inches of the floor, making sure your body is in a straight line from your head to your knees. Try not to flare your elbows to the sides.

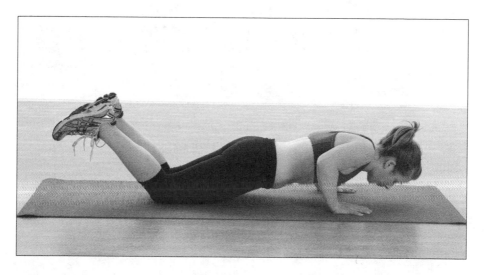

**2** Raise your body to the starting position by pushing up with your arms. The movement should be smooth and controlled.

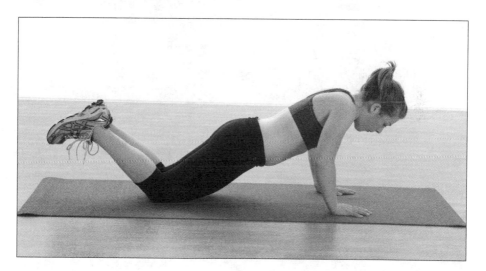

# Knee push-up with knuckles

*If you find knee push-ups hurt your wrists, you can do them with your knuckles instead. Don't worry, knuckle push-ups are not just for the hard-core push-up folks! A surprising number of people experience wrist discomfort as they perform "good-form" push-ups, but by closing your hands and making a fist, your body weight ends up on your knuckles instead of your palms, thus avoiding the wrist extension motion.*

**STARTING POSITION:** Assume a comfortable kneeling position on the floor. Make fists with your hands and place your knuckles directly on a rolled-up towel or padded exercise mat directly under your chest. Maintain a straight line from your shoulders to your feet by keeping your abs tight. Do not raise your butt in the air or allow your back to sag to the ground.

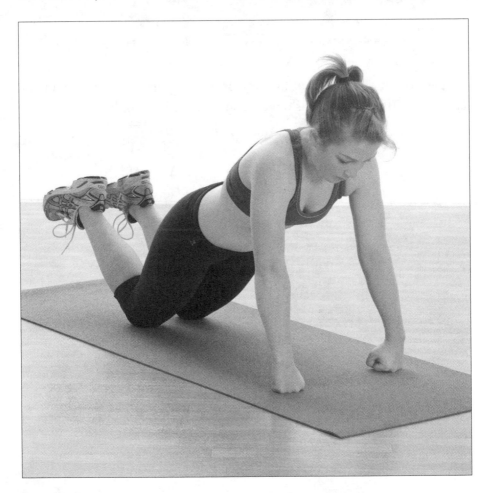

**1** Breathe in as you lower your torso to the ground, stopping when your elbows form a 90-degree angle and your chest is an inch or two from the ground.

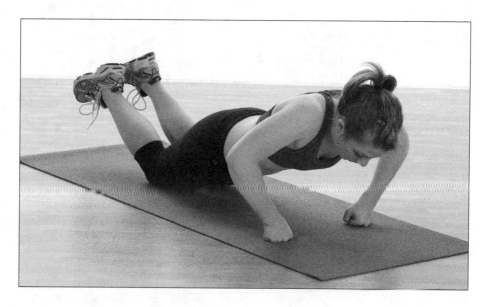

**2** Breathe out as you push yourself up using your arms. Think of raising yourself by attempting to push the ground away from you. The power for the push will predominantly come from your shoulders and chest. The movement should be smooth and controlled.

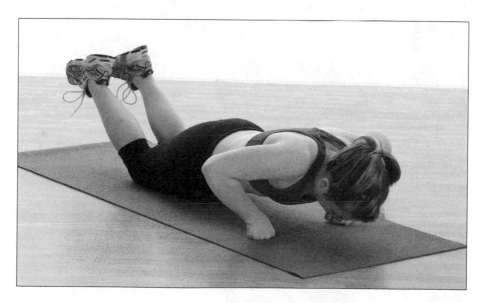

# 7 WEEKS TO 100 PUSH-UPS LOG

| WEEK | DAY | SET 1 | | SET 2 | | SET 3 | | SET 4 | | SET 5 | | SET 6 | | SET 7 | | SET 8 | | TOTAL | MAX |
|---|---|---|---|---|---|---|---|---|---|---|---|---|---|---|---|---|---|---|---|
| | | Goal | Actual | Goal | Actual | Goal | Actual | Goal | Actual | Goal | Actual | Goal | Actual | Goal | Actual | Goal | Actual | | |
| **1** | M | | | | | | | | | | | | | | | | | | |
| | W | | | | | | | | | | | | | | | | | | |
| | F | | | | | | | | | | | | | | | | | | |
| WEEKLY TOTAL | | | | | | | | | | | | | | | | | | | |
| **2** | M | | | | | | | | | | | | | | | | | | |
| | W | | | | | | | | | | | | | | | | | | |
| | F | | | | | | | | | | | | | | | | | | |
| WEEKLY TOTAL | | | | | | | | | | | | | | | | | | | |
| **3** | M | | | | | | | | | | | | | | | | | | |
| | W | | | | | | | | | | | | | | | | | | |
| | F | | | | | | | | | | | | | | | | | | |
| WEEKLY TOTAL | | | | | | | | | | | | | | | | | | | |
| **4** | M | | | | | | | | | | | | | | | | | | |
| | W | | | | | | | | | | | | | | | | | | |
| | F | | | | | | | | | | | | | | | | | | |
| WEEKLY TOTAL | | | | | | | | | | | | | | | | | | | |
| **5** | M | | | | | | | | | | | | | | | | | | |
| | W | | | | | | | | | | | | | | | | | | |
| | F | | | | | | | | | | | | | | | | | | |
| WEEKLY TOTAL | | | | | | | | | | | | | | | | | | | |

# 7 WEEKS TO 100 PUSH-UPS LOG

| WEEK | DAY | SET 1 | | SET 2 | | SET 3 | | SET 4 | | SET 5 | | SET 6 | | SET 7 | | SET 8 | | TOTAL | MAX |
|---|---|---|---|---|---|---|---|---|---|---|---|---|---|---|---|---|---|---|---|
| | | Goal | Actual | Goal | Actual | Goal | Actual | Goal | Actual | Goal | Actual | Goal | Actual | Goal | Actual | Goal | Actual | | |
| **6** | M | | | | | | | | | | | | | | | | | | |
| | W | | | | | | | | | | | | | | | | | | |
| | F | | | | | | | | | | | | | | | | | | |
| WEEKLY TOTAL | | | | | | | | | | | | | | | | | | | |
| **7** | M | | | | | | | | | | | | | | | | | | |
| | W | | | | | | | | | | | | | | | | | | |
| | F | | | | | | | | | | | | | | | | | | |
| WEEKLY TOTAL | | | | | | | | | | | | | | | | | | | |
| **8** | M | | | | | | | | | | | | | | | | | | |
| | W | | | | | | | | | | | | | | | | | | |
| | F | | | | | | | | | | | | | | | | | | |
| WEEKLY TOTAL | | | | | | | | | | | | | | | | | | | |
| **9** | M | | | | | | | | | | | | | | | | | | |
| | W | | | | | | | | | | | | | | | | | | |
| | F | | | | | | | | | | | | | | | | | | |
| WEEKLY TOTAL | | | | | | | | | | | | | | | | | | | |
| **10** | M | | | | | | | | | | | | | | | | | | |
| | W | | | | | | | | | | | | | | | | | | |
| | F | | | | | | | | | | | | | | | | | | |
| WEEKLY TOTAL | | | | | | | | | | | | | | | | | | | |
| GRAND TOTAL | | | | | | | | | | | | | | | | | | | |

# 7 WEEKS TO 100 PUSH-UPS LOG

| WEEK | DAY | SET 1 | | SET 2 | | SET 3 | | SET 4 | | SET 5 | | SET 6 | | SET 7 | | SET 8 | | TOTAL | MAX |
|---|---|---|---|---|---|---|---|---|---|---|---|---|---|---|---|---|---|---|---|
| | | Goal | Actual | Goal | Actual | Goal | Actual | Goal | Actual | Goal | Actual | Goal | Actual | Goal | Actual | Goal | Actual | | |
| **1** | M | | | | | | | | | | | | | | | | | | |
| | W | | | | | | | | | | | | | | | | | | |
| | F | | | | | | | | | | | | | | | | | | |
| | WEEKLY TOTAL | | | | | | | | | | | | | | | | | | |
| **2** | M | | | | | | | | | | | | | | | | | | |
| | W | | | | | | | | | | | | | | | | | | |
| | F | | | | | | | | | | | | | | | | | | |
| | WEEKLY TOTAL | | | | | | | | | | | | | | | | | | |
| **3** | M | | | | | | | | | | | | | | | | | | |
| | W | | | | | | | | | | | | | | | | | | |
| | F | | | | | | | | | | | | | | | | | | |
| | WEEKLY TOTAL | | | | | | | | | | | | | | | | | | |
| **4** | M | | | | | | | | | | | | | | | | | | |
| | W | | | | | | | | | | | | | | | | | | |
| | F | | | | | | | | | | | | | | | | | | |
| | WEEKLY TOTAL | | | | | | | | | | | | | | | | | | |
| **5** | M | | | | | | | | | | | | | | | | | | |
| | W | | | | | | | | | | | | | | | | | | |
| | F | | | | | | | | | | | | | | | | | | |
| | WEEKLY TOTAL | | | | | | | | | | | | | | | | | | |

# 7 WEEKS TO 100 PUSH-UPS LOG

| WEEK | DAY | SET 1 Goal | SET 1 Actual | SET 2 Goal | SET 2 Actual | SET 3 Goal | SET 3 Actual | SET 4 Goal | SET 4 Actual | SET 5 Goal | SET 5 Actual | SET 6 Goal | SET 6 Actual | SET 7 Goal | SET 7 Actual | SET 8 Goal | SET 8 Actual | TOTAL | MAX |
|------|-----|------|------|------|------|------|------|------|------|------|------|------|------|------|------|------|------|-------|-----|
| 6 | M | | | | | | | | | | | | | | | | | | |
| 6 | W | | | | | | | | | | | | | | | | | | |
| 6 | F | | | | | | | | | | | | | | | | | | |
| WEEKLY TOTAL | | | | | | | | | | | | | | | | | | | |
| 7 | M | | | | | | | | | | | | | | | | | | |
| 7 | W | | | | | | | | | | | | | | | | | | |
| 7 | F | | | | | | | | | | | | | | | | | | |
| WEEKLY TOTAL | | | | | | | | | | | | | | | | | | | |
| 8 | M | | | | | | | | | | | | | | | | | | |
| 8 | W | | | | | | | | | | | | | | | | | | |
| 8 | F | | | | | | | | | | | | | | | | | | |
| WEEKLY TOTAL | | | | | | | | | | | | | | | | | | | |
| 9 | M | | | | | | | | | | | | | | | | | | |
| 9 | W | | | | | | | | | | | | | | | | | | |
| 9 | F | | | | | | | | | | | | | | | | | | |
| WEEKLY TOTAL | | | | | | | | | | | | | | | | | | | |
| 10 | M | | | | | | | | | | | | | | | | | | |
| 10 | W | | | | | | | | | | | | | | | | | | |
| 10 | F | | | | | | | | | | | | | | | | | | |
| WEEKLY TOTAL | | | | | | | | | | | | | | | | | | | |
| GRAND TOTAL | | | | | | | | | | | | | | | | | | | |

# 7 WEEKS TO 100 PUSH-UPS LOG

| WEEK | DAY | SET 1 | | SET 2 | | SET 3 | | SET 4 | | SET 5 | | SET 6 | | SET 7 | | SET 8 | | TOTAL | MAX |
|---|---|---|---|---|---|---|---|---|---|---|---|---|---|---|---|---|---|---|---|
| | | Goal | Actual | Goal | Actual | Goal | Actual | Goal | Actual | Goal | Actual | Goal | Actual | Goal | Actual | Goal | Actual | | |
| **1** | M | | | | | | | | | | | | | | | | | | |
| | W | | | | | | | | | | | | | | | | | | |
| | F | | | | | | | | | | | | | | | | | | |
| | WEEKLY TOTAL | | | | | | | | | | | | | | | | | | |
| **2** | M | | | | | | | | | | | | | | | | | | |
| | W | | | | | | | | | | | | | | | | | | |
| | F | | | | | | | | | | | | | | | | | | |
| | WEEKLY TOTAL | | | | | | | | | | | | | | | | | | |
| **3** | M | | | | | | | | | | | | | | | | | | |
| | W | | | | | | | | | | | | | | | | | | |
| | F | | | | | | | | | | | | | | | | | | |
| | WEEKLY TOTAL | | | | | | | | | | | | | | | | | | |
| **4** | M | | | | | | | | | | | | | | | | | | |
| | W | | | | | | | | | | | | | | | | | | |
| | F | | | | | | | | | | | | | | | | | | |
| | WEEKLY TOTAL | | | | | | | | | | | | | | | | | | |
| **5** | M | | | | | | | | | | | | | | | | | | |
| | W | | | | | | | | | | | | | | | | | | |
| | F | | | | | | | | | | | | | | | | | | |
| | WEEKLY TOTAL | | | | | | | | | | | | | | | | | | |

# 7 WEEKS TO 100 PUSH-UPS LOG

| WEEK | DAY | SET 1 | | SET 2 | | SET 3 | | SET 4 | | SET 5 | | SET 6 | | SET 7 | | SET 8 | | TOTAL | MAX |
|---|---|---|---|---|---|---|---|---|---|---|---|---|---|---|---|---|---|---|---|
| | | Goal | Actual | Goal | Actual | Goal | Actual | Goal | Actual | Goal | Actual | Goal | Actual | Goal | Actual | Goal | Actual | | |
| **6** | M | | | | | | | | | | | | | | | | | | |
| | W | | | | | | | | | | | | | | | | | | |
| | F | | | | | | | | | | | | | | | | | | |
| WEEKLY TOTAL | | | | | | | | | | | | | | | | | | | |
| **7** | M | | | | | | | | | | | | | | | | | | |
| | W | | | | | | | | | | | | | | | | | | |
| | F | | | | | | | | | | | | | | | | | | |
| WEEKLY TOTAL | | | | | | | | | | | | | | | | | | | |
| **8** | M | | | | | | | | | | | | | | | | | | |
| | W | | | | | | | | | | | | | | | | | | |
| | F | | | | | | | | | | | | | | | | | | |
| WEEKLY TOTAL | | | | | | | | | | | | | | | | | | | |
| **9** | M | | | | | | | | | | | | | | | | | | |
| | W | | | | | | | | | | | | | | | | | | |
| | F | | | | | | | | | | | | | | | | | | |
| WEEKLY TOTAL | | | | | | | | | | | | | | | | | | | |
| **10** | M | | | | | | | | | | | | | | | | | | |
| | W | | | | | | | | | | | | | | | | | | |
| | F | | | | | | | | | | | | | | | | | | |
| WEEKLY TOTAL | | | | | | | | | | | | | | | | | | | |
| GRAND TOTAL | | | | | | | | | | | | | | | | | | | |

# 7 WEEKS TO 100 PUSH-UPS LOG

| WEEK | DAY | SET 1 | | SET 2 | | SET 3 | | SET 4 | | SET 5 | | SET 6 | | SET 7 | | SET 8 | | TOTAL | MAX |
|---|---|---|---|---|---|---|---|---|---|---|---|---|---|---|---|---|---|---|---|
| | | Goal | Actual | Goal | Actual | Goal | Actual | Goal | Actual | Goal | Actual | Goal | Actual | Goal | Actual | Goal | Actual | | |
| **1** | M | | | | | | | | | | | | | | | | | | |
| | W | | | | | | | | | | | | | | | | | | |
| | F | | | | | | | | | | | | | | | | | | |
| | WEEKLY TOTAL | | | | | | | | | | | | | | | | | | |
| **2** | M | | | | | | | | | | | | | | | | | | |
| | W | | | | | | | | | | | | | | | | | | |
| | F | | | | | | | | | | | | | | | | | | |
| | WEEKLY TOTAL | | | | | | | | | | | | | | | | | | |
| **3** | M | | | | | | | | | | | | | | | | | | |
| | W | | | | | | | | | | | | | | | | | | |
| | F | | | | | | | | | | | | | | | | | | |
| | WEEKLY TOTAL | | | | | | | | | | | | | | | | | | |
| **4** | M | | | | | | | | | | | | | | | | | | |
| | W | | | | | | | | | | | | | | | | | | |
| | F | | | | | | | | | | | | | | | | | | |
| | WEEKLY TOTAL | | | | | | | | | | | | | | | | | | |
| **5** | M | | | | | | | | | | | | | | | | | | |
| | W | | | | | | | | | | | | | | | | | | |
| | F | | | | | | | | | | | | | | | | | | |
| | WEEKLY TOTAL | | | | | | | | | | | | | | | | | | |

# 7 WEEKS TO 100 PUSH-UPS LOG

| WEEK | DAY | SET 1 | | SET 2 | | SET 3 | | SET 4 | | SET 5 | | SET 6 | | SET 7 | | SET 8 | | TOTAL | MAX |
|------|-----|-------|---|-------|---|-------|---|-------|---|-------|---|-------|---|-------|---|-------|---|-------|-----|
| | | Goal | Actual | Goal | Actual | Goal | Actual | Goal | Actual | Goal | Actual | Goal | Actual | Goal | Actual | Goal | Actual | | |
| **6** | M | | | | | | | | | | | | | | | | | | |
| | W | | | | | | | | | | | | | | | | | | |
| | F | | | | | | | | | | | | | | | | | | |
| WEEKLY TOTAL | | | | | | | | | | | | | | | | | | | |
| **7** | M | | | | | | | | | | | | | | | | | | |
| | W | | | | | | | | | | | | | | | | | | |
| | F | | | | | | | | | | | | | | | | | | |
| WEEKLY TOTAL | | | | | | | | | | | | | | | | | | | |
| **8** | M | | | | | | | | | | | | | | | | | | |
| | W | | | | | | | | | | | | | | | | | | |
| | F | | | | | | | | | | | | | | | | | | |
| WEEKLY TOTAL | | | | | | | | | | | | | | | | | | | |
| **9** | M | | | | | | | | | | | | | | | | | | |
| | W | | | | | | | | | | | | | | | | | | |
| | F | | | | | | | | | | | | | | | | | | |
| WEEKLY TOTAL | | | | | | | | | | | | | | | | | | | |
| **10** | M | | | | | | | | | | | | | | | | | | |
| | W | | | | | | | | | | | | | | | | | | |
| | F | | | | | | | | | | | | | | | | | | |
| WEEKLY TOTAL | | | | | | | | | | | | | | | | | | | |
| GRAND TOTAL | | | | | | | | | | | | | | | | | | | |

# 7 WEEKS TO 100 PUSH-UPS LOG

| WEEK | DAY | SET 1 | | SET 2 | | SET 3 | | SET 4 | | SET 5 | | SET 6 | | SET 7 | | SET 8 | | TOTAL | MAX |
|------|-----|------|--------|------|--------|------|--------|------|--------|------|--------|------|--------|------|--------|------|--------|-------|-----|
| | | Goal | Actual | Goal | Actual | Goal | Actual | Goal | Actual | Goal | Actual | Goal | Actual | Goal | Actual | Goal | Actual | | |
| **1** | M | | | | | | | | | | | | | | | | | | |
| | W | | | | | | | | | | | | | | | | | | |
| | F | | | | | | | | | | | | | | | | | | |
| | WEEKLY TOTAL | | | | | | | | | | | | | | | | | | |
| **2** | M | | | | | | | | | | | | | | | | | | |
| | W | | | | | | | | | | | | | | | | | | |
| | F | | | | | | | | | | | | | | | | | | |
| | WEEKLY TOTAL | | | | | | | | | | | | | | | | | | |
| **3** | M | | | | | | | | | | | | | | | | | | |
| | W | | | | | | | | | | | | | | | | | | |
| | F | | | | | | | | | | | | | | | | | | |
| | WEEKLY TOTAL | | | | | | | | | | | | | | | | | | |
| **4** | M | | | | | | | | | | | | | | | | | | |
| | W | | | | | | | | | | | | | | | | | | |
| | F | | | | | | | | | | | | | | | | | | |
| | WEEKLY TOTAL | | | | | | | | | | | | | | | | | | |
| **5** | M | | | | | | | | | | | | | | | | | | |
| | W | | | | | | | | | | | | | | | | | | |
| | F | | | | | | | | | | | | | | | | | | |
| | WEEKLY TOTAL | | | | | | | | | | | | | | | | | | |

# 7 WEEKS TO 100 PUSH-UPS LOG

| WEEK | DAY | SET 1 | | SET 2 | | SET 3 | | SET 4 | | SET 5 | | SET 6 | | SET 7 | | SET 8 | | TOTAL | MAX |
|---|---|---|---|---|---|---|---|---|---|---|---|---|---|---|---|---|---|---|---|
| | | Goal | Actual | Goal | Actual | Goal | Actual | Goal | Actual | Goal | Actual | Goal | Actual | Goal | Actual | Goal | Actual | | |
| **6** | M | | | | | | | | | | | | | | | | | | |
| | W | | | | | | | | | | | | | | | | | | |
| | F | | | | | | | | | | | | | | | | | | |
| WEEKLY TOTAL | | | | | | | | | | | | | | | | | | | |
| **7** | M | | | | | | | | | | | | | | | | | | |
| | W | | | | | | | | | | | | | | | | | | |
| | F | | | | | | | | | | | | | | | | | | |
| WEEKLY TOTAL | | | | | | | | | | | | | | | | | | | |
| **8** | M | | | | | | | | | | | | | | | | | | |
| | W | | | | | | | | | | | | | | | | | | |
| | F | | | | | | | | | | | | | | | | | | |
| WEEKLY TOTAL | | | | | | | | | | | | | | | | | | | |
| **9** | M | | | | | | | | | | | | | | | | | | |
| | W | | | | | | | | | | | | | | | | | | |
| | F | | | | | | | | | | | | | | | | | | |
| WEEKLY TOTAL | | | | | | | | | | | | | | | | | | | |
| **10** | M | | | | | | | | | | | | | | | | | | |
| | W | | | | | | | | | | | | | | | | | | |
| | F | | | | | | | | | | | | | | | | | | |
| WEEKLY TOTAL | | | | | | | | | | | | | | | | | | | |
| GRAND TOTAL | | | | | | | | | | | | | | | | | | | |

# 7 WEEKS TO 100 PUSH-UPS LOG

| WEEK | DAY | SET 1 | | SET 2 | | SET 3 | | SET 4 | | SET 5 | | SET 6 | | SET 7 | | SET 8 | | TOTAL | MAX |
|---|---|---|---|---|---|---|---|---|---|---|---|---|---|---|---|---|---|---|---|
| | | Goal | Actual | Goal | Actual | Goal | Actual | Goal | Actual | Goal | Actual | Goal | Actual | Goal | Actual | Goal | Actual | | |
| **1** | M | | | | | | | | | | | | | | | | | | |
| | W | | | | | | | | | | | | | | | | | | |
| | F | | | | | | | | | | | | | | | | | | |
| | WEEKLY TOTAL | | | | | | | | | | | | | | | | | | |
| **2** | M | | | | | | | | | | | | | | | | | | |
| | W | | | | | | | | | | | | | | | | | | |
| | F | | | | | | | | | | | | | | | | | | |
| | WEEKLY TOTAL | | | | | | | | | | | | | | | | | | |
| **3** | M | | | | | | | | | | | | | | | | | | |
| | W | | | | | | | | | | | | | | | | | | |
| | F | | | | | | | | | | | | | | | | | | |
| | WEEKLY TOTAL | | | | | | | | | | | | | | | | | | |
| **4** | M | | | | | | | | | | | | | | | | | | |
| | W | | | | | | | | | | | | | | | | | | |
| | F | | | | | | | | | | | | | | | | | | |
| | WEEKLY TOTAL | | | | | | | | | | | | | | | | | | |
| **5** | M | | | | | | | | | | | | | | | | | | |
| | W | | | | | | | | | | | | | | | | | | |
| | F | | | | | | | | | | | | | | | | | | |
| | WEEKLY TOTAL | | | | | | | | | | | | | | | | | | |

# 7 WEEKS TO 100 PUSH-UPS LOG

| WEEK | DAY | SET 1 | | SET 2 | | SET 3 | | SET 4 | | SET 5 | | SET 6 | | SET 7 | | SET 8 | | TOTAL | MAX |
|------|-----|-------|---|-------|---|-------|---|-------|---|-------|---|-------|---|-------|---|-------|---|-------|-----|
| | | Goal | Actual | Goal | Actual | Goal | Actual | Goal | Actual | Goal | Actual | Goal | Actual | Goal | Actual | Goal | Actual | | |
| **6** | M | | | | | | | | | | | | | | | | | | |
| | W | | | | | | | | | | | | | | | | | | |
| | F | | | | | | | | | | | | | | | | | | |
| WEEKLY TOTAL | | | | | | | | | | | | | | | | | | | |
| **7** | M | | | | | | | | | | | | | | | | | | |
| | W | | | | | | | | | | | | | | | | | | |
| | F | | | | | | | | | | | | | | | | | | |
| WEEKLY TOTAL | | | | | | | | | | | | | | | | | | | |
| **8** | M | | | | | | | | | | | | | | | | | | |
| | W | | | | | | | | | | | | | | | | | | |
| | F | | | | | | | | | | | | | | | | | | |
| WEEKLY TOTAL | | | | | | | | | | | | | | | | | | | |
| **9** | M | | | | | | | | | | | | | | | | | | |
| | W | | | | | | | | | | | | | | | | | | |
| | F | | | | | | | | | | | | | | | | | | |
| WEEKLY TOTAL | | | | | | | | | | | | | | | | | | | |
| **10** | M | | | | | | | | | | | | | | | | | | |
| | W | | | | | | | | | | | | | | | | | | |
| | F | | | | | | | | | | | | | | | | | | |
| WEEKLY TOTAL | | | | | | | | | | | | | | | | | | | |
| GRAND TOTAL | | | | | | | | | | | | | | | | | | | |

# PRELIMINARY PROGRAM PUSH-UPS LOG

| WEEK | DAY | SET 1 | | SET 2 | | SET 3 | | SET 4 | | SET 5 | | SET 6 | | SET 7 | | SET 8 | | TOTAL | MAX |
|---|---|---|---|---|---|---|---|---|---|---|---|---|---|---|---|---|---|---|---|
| | | Goal | Actual | Goal | Actual | Goal | Actual | Goal | Actual | Goal | Actual | Goal | Actual | Goal | Actual | Goal | Actual | | |
| **1** | M | | | | | | | | | | | | | | | | | | |
| | W | | | | | | | | | | | | | | | | | | |
| | F | | | | | | | | | | | | | | | | | | |
| WEEKLY TOTAL | | | | | | | | | | | | | | | | | | | |
| **2** | M | | | | | | | | | | | | | | | | | | |
| | W | | | | | | | | | | | | | | | | | | |
| | F | | | | | | | | | | | | | | | | | | |
| WEEKLY TOTAL | | | | | | | | | | | | | | | | | | | |
| **3** | M | | | | | | | | | | | | | | | | | | |
| | W | | | | | | | | | | | | | | | | | | |
| | F | | | | | | | | | | | | | | | | | | |
| WEEKLY TOTAL | | | | | | | | | | | | | | | | | | | |
| **4** | M | | | | | | | | | | | | | | | | | | |
| | W | | | | | | | | | | | | | | | | | | |
| | F | | | | | | | | | | | | | | | | | | |
| WEEKLY TOTAL | | | | | | | | | | | | | | | | | | | |
| GRAND TOTAL | | | | | | | | | | | | | | | | | | | |

# PRELIMINARY PROGRAM PUSH-UPS LOG

| WEEK | DAY | SET 1 | | SET 2 | | SET 3 | | SET 4 | | SET 5 | | SET 6 | | SET 7 | | SET 8 | | TOTAL | MAX |
|---|---|---|---|---|---|---|---|---|---|---|---|---|---|---|---|---|---|---|---|
| | | Goal | Actual | Goal | Actual | Goal | Actual | Goal | Actual | Goal | Actual | Goal | Actual | Goal | Actual | Goal | Actual | | |
| **1** | M | | | | | | | | | | | | | | | | | | |
| | W | | | | | | | | | | | | | | | | | | |
| | F | | | | | | | | | | | | | | | | | | |
| WEEKLY TOTAL | | | | | | | | | | | | | | | | | | | |
| **2** | M | | | | | | | | | | | | | | | | | | |
| | W | | | | | | | | | | | | | | | | | | |
| | F | | | | | | | | | | | | | | | | | | |
| WEEKLY TOTAL | | | | | | | | | | | | | | | | | | | |
| **3** | M | | | | | | | | | | | | | | | | | | |
| | W | | | | | | | | | | | | | | | | | | |
| | F | | | | | | | | | | | | | | | | | | |
| WEEKLY TOTAL | | | | | | | | | | | | | | | | | | | |
| **4** | M | | | | | | | | | | | | | | | | | | |
| | W | | | | | | | | | | | | | | | | | | |
| | F | | | | | | | | | | | | | | | | | | |
| WEEKLY TOTAL | | | | | | | | | | | | | | | | | | | |
| GRAND TOTAL | | | | | | | | | | | | | | | | | | | |

# PRELIMINARY PROGRAM PUSH-UPS LOG

| WEEK | DAY | SET 1 | | SET 2 | | SET 3 | | SET 4 | | SET 5 | | SET 6 | | SET 7 | | SET 8 | | TOTAL | MAX |
|---|---|---|---|---|---|---|---|---|---|---|---|---|---|---|---|---|---|---|---|
| | | Goal | Actual | Goal | Actual | Goal | Actual | Goal | Actual | Goal | Actual | Goal | Actual | Goal | Actual | Goal | Actual | | |
| **1** | M | | | | | | | | | | | | | | | | | | |
| | W | | | | | | | | | | | | | | | | | | |
| | F | | | | | | | | | | | | | | | | | | |
| | WEEKLY TOTAL | | | | | | | | | | | | | | | | | | |
| **2** | M | | | | | | | | | | | | | | | | | | |
| | W | | | | | | | | | | | | | | | | | | |
| | F | | | | | | | | | | | | | | | | | | |
| | WEEKLY TOTAL | | | | | | | | | | | | | | | | | | |
| **3** | M | | | | | | | | | | | | | | | | | | |
| | W | | | | | | | | | | | | | | | | | | |
| | F | | | | | | | | | | | | | | | | | | |
| | WEEKLY TOTAL | | | | | | | | | | | | | | | | | | |
| **4** | M | | | | | | | | | | | | | | | | | | |
| | W | | | | | | | | | | | | | | | | | | |
| | F | | | | | | | | | | | | | | | | | | |
| | WEEKLY TOTAL | | | | | | | | | | | | | | | | | | |
| GRAND TOTAL | | | | | | | | | | | | | | | | | | | |

# Index

# Acknowledgments

It takes far more than an author to write a book, so I shall do my best to thank everyone who helped with this one. Thanks to Nick Denton-Brown, acquisitions editor at Ulysses Press, for the initial contact and guiding hand through the early stages of development. Without his vision, there would simply be no book.

Thanks also to Lily Chou, Ulysses Press fitness book editor, for expertly orchestrating the transformation of a dream into a reality. Her positive feedback, excellent suggestions, and expertise have been invaluable.

There are numerous online fitness friends to thank, too, many of whom offered fantastic advice and recommendations based on years of exercise experience.

And then, of course, there are the friends, colleagues, and family members who have inspired and supported me throughout. I am very fortunate to know so many wonderful people.

Finally, and I've saved the most important for last—thank you, Ally, for your patience, support, and love, and for allowing me the opportunity to explore many new avenues.

# About the Author

Born in Wales but now living on the East Coast of the U.S., **STEVE SPEIRS** is an avid runner and fitness enthusiast. Since entering his first race in the early 1980s, he has been hooked on an active lifestyle and is always seeking new challenges and the next level of fitness.

Competing in numerous races a year, Speirs has completed 60+ marathons and over 75 ultramarathons with a 100-mile best of 15:26:25.

Speirs is a proud son, husband, brother, and father, and dedicates *7 Weeks to 100 Push-Ups* to his ever-supportive family.